How to Improve at Fitness and Beat the Competition:
Sport and Exercise Science for Athletes in Search of Excellence

Powered by:

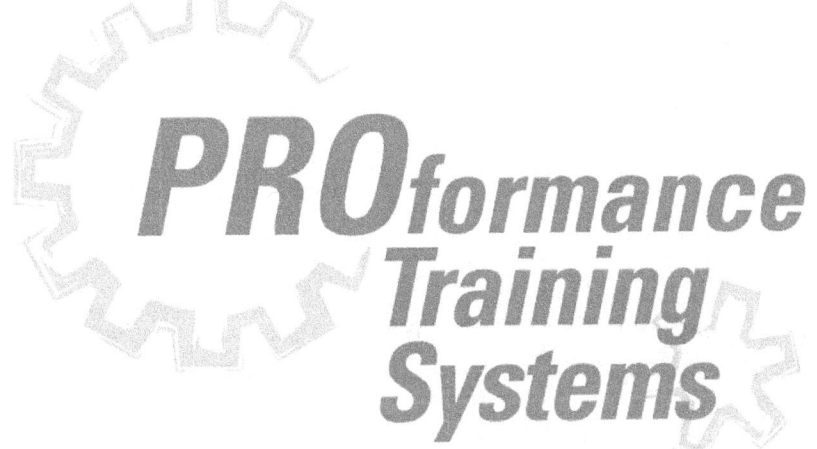

Christopher P. Johnson

FIRST EDITION

PROformance, LLC. 1st ed.: Newton, Massachusetts.

Includes bibliography references.

ISBN 9781537286150
ISBN: 1537286153
Library of Congress Control Number: 2018901696
CreateSpace Independent Publishing Platform, North Charleston, SC

No portion of this book is meant to be or should be taken as medical advice. I am not a medical doctor, and any exercise or nutritional program should be cleared by a medical doctor prior to beginning.

To Mom and Dad and my beautiful wife Stephanie.

Other Works by Christopher Johnson

PR Pace: Strength and Performance Training for Distance Runners

Leadership Development Method: A literature review of leadership development strategy and tactics

Gamification in Adventure and Wilderness Sports: A literature review of game-based mechanic's ability to increase attraction, engagement, and retention in outdoor sports

More information can be found on Christopher Johnson at www.improvewithchris.com

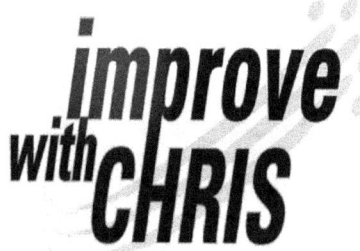

Contents

Acknowledgments

This book is the accumulation of years of research and coaching experience. Not only my research, but the research of others. I have simply gathered what I feel is some of the most useful research from sport and exercise science and put it into a collection of essays. The scientist who came before me did the heavy lifting, all I did was filter through their hard work to develop PROformance Training Systems, which has allowed me to coach hundreds of athletes towards excellence over the years and I am now sharing with you. It is for this reason I chose a baton exchange between runners as my cover image. The baton exchange symbolizes the passing along of knowledge and experience. All I have done is bind their lessons in a convenient book. This book is also a product of the coaches who have shared their wisdom with me over the years. Every athlete should have a great coach behind them, and I am grateful to have had decades of coaching experience shared with me.

Thank You Coaches

Bold Lines

As you read this book, you will notice **bold lines** throughout the chapters. These bold lines act as cliff notes. They are quick one liners aimed to help you digest the science as well as act as a brief summary. The bold lines are placed after their relevant section, so if one of them catches your eye, read the above section. A collection of the bold lines is also included in Appendix B at the end of the book.

Bold Lines Act as Cliff Notes

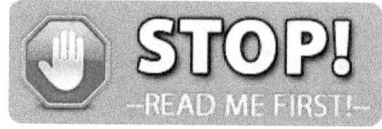

PROformance Training Systems

Anyone reading this book is excited to improve and is looking for the best sport-and-exercise science, unwilling to waste time with unjustified trends. Yet, when looking around a fitness center, I often see people focusing on components of fitness with no direction or method. Thousands of athletes are training for their sport with the desire to improve but are lacking proper guidance. With that said, I want to start this collection of essays with what PROformance Training Systems (PTS) is and how to employ the system, and then we will dive into the science of why it should be your athlete training system of choice.

The following essays explain or support the principles behind PTS. By learning the science of why and how something works, it allows you to modify the system to your needs. Even though PTS is a highly encompassing system, modifications may be necessary to meet peculiar goals. I refer to PTS as *systems* rather than a *system* as a reminder that excellence cannot be achieved with a single answer or particular discipline, but rather the best combination of resources and insight for the individual. A good coach knows the popular training methods for a sport or position, but a great coach takes into account their athlete's individual needs, abilities, and desires.

It is my hope that PROformance Training Systems grants you insight into how to effectively tailor a sport and exercise training program allowing you to achieve excellence. There are hundreds of training programs out there, PTS teaches you how and when to use them by showing you the proper stages or as I refer to them "themes" of athletic progression. Allowing you or your coach to develop a master plan to attain your goal.

I strongly encourage all athletes, novice or veteran, to get medical clearance before beginning a new exercise program. It is also in my opinion that every athlete has a coach to guide him through his journey. Regardless of how many years of experience you may have, everyone can gain something from a mentor. Remember, the best athletes in the world have coaches.

PROformance Training Systems Teaches You How to Organize Training Methods

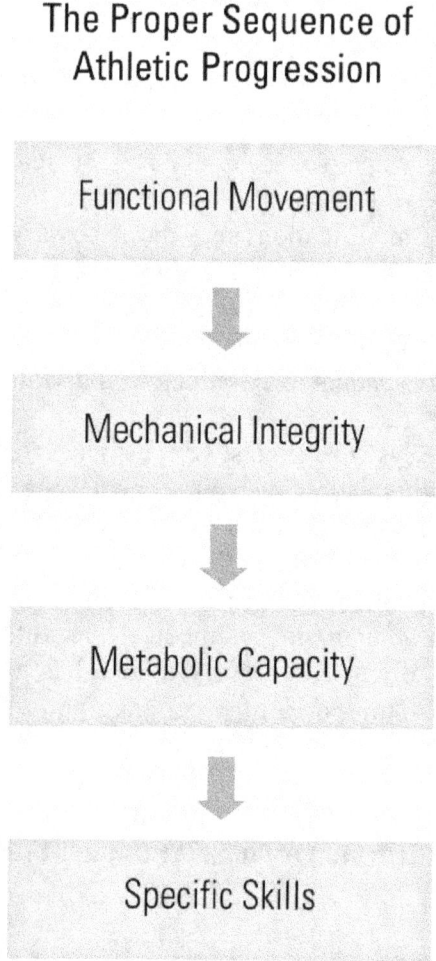

The Proper Sequence of Athletic Progression

Functional Movement

↓

Mechanical Integrity

↓

Metabolic Capacity

↓

Specific Skills

When it comes to improving ourselves as athletes, the appropriate steps should be taken in the correct sequence. These steps are functional movement, mechanical integrity, metabolic capacity, and specific skills in that order. Functional movement is the ability to move the body through basic practical movement patterns properly without pain. This step should not be viewed as exercise but rather as learning. If we want to advance toward athletic excellence, we must first learn the proper functional movements and be able to complete them free of pain.

The second step is mechanical integrity. Once correct movement patterns are put in place, the mechanical structures of the body (muscles, tendon, ligaments, and fascia) must be fortified. Heavy and intense resistance training should not be performed without first establishing mechanical integrity. Moreover, it would not make sense to progress someone toward cardiovascular fitness if his body is not ready to handle the stress of the associated workload. Therefore, adequate time must be taken to ensure appropriate mechanical integrity prior to implementing the repetitive movements and high-volume loads associated with cardiovascular training.

Next, metabolic capacity can be established. The metabolic pathways can be anaerobic or aerobic in nature; they are the phosphagen system (anaerobic), glycolysis (anaerobic), or aerobic system (aerobic). Proper metabolic pathways should be trained for each sport. Olympic-lifting energy pathways are very different from distance running. Therefore, they should be handled differently; however, each discipline should be developed with equal importance.

Phosphagen & Glycolysis = Anaerobic; Aerobic = With Oxygen

Finally, specific skills can be developed. To truly master and excel in a specific sporting skill, one must first acquire ample functional movement, structural integrity, and metabolic capacity associated with that skill. Always reassessing progress, making certain one does not develop a weakness in one area by focusing too strongly on any one theme. Skipping or overemphasizing any one of these steps will only set you up for injury or suboptimal performance.

Skills training should be taught using the "crawl, walk, run" method. This entails starting small and slow, gradually adding more when applicable until skills can be performed properly at full speed and integrated into movement drills, plyometrics, and high intensity interval training (HIIT). If you are experiencing difficulty learning a skill, break it down "by the numbers." By the numbers is a learning technique when you break a skill down into smaller parts, each part numbered as steps in the entire process. Then act out all of the steps in order by the numbers.

For optimal athleticism to be achieved, the proper sequence of athletic progression must be followed. Just as you cannot win a war without an army, cannot have an army without soldiers, and cannot have soldiers without proper training and tools, the body cannot reach its athletic potential without first attaining specific skills, it cannot reach the skills without the metabolic capacity to perform, it can't perform without the structural integrity to hold it all together allowing it to move, and it can't move correctly and efficiently if it does not have proper movement patterns and stability. Follow the proper sequence of athletic progression shown on the next page and ensure optimal performance.

Athletes Need to Progress in The Proper Sequence to Reach Their True Potential

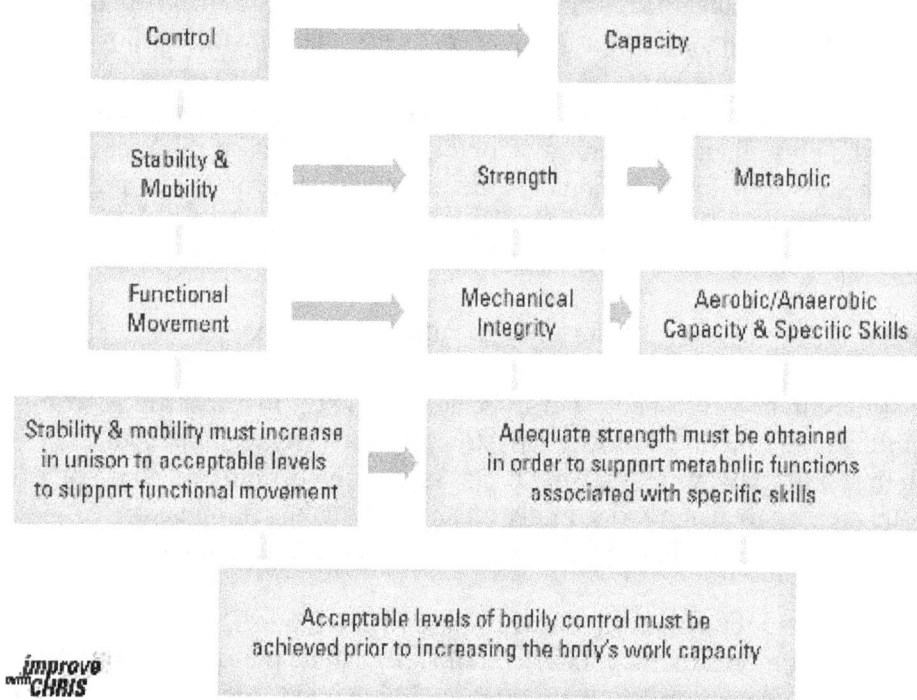

Above is a diagram laying out how an athlete should progress their training. The flowchart should be read top to bottom and left to right.

Excellence is reaching the pinnacle of a discipline and mastering all the steps along the way. Achieving excellence in human performance is built on solid foundations. The roots of these foundations are control and capacity. Control is the body's ability to adequately manage itself through sufficiently and simultaneously limiting and allowing motion. Capacity, on the other hand, is the ability to elevate the body to heightened levels of control. Efficient control must be obtained prior to increasing capacity to support the repetitive nature of metabolic functions associated with specific skills development while avoiding injury due to muscle imbalances and poor arthrokinematics (joint movement) that can be amplified during repetitive movements (i.e., high-volume training). The basis of control is stability and mobility. Stability is the product of proprioception (the body's self-awareness in space) and timing (properly adjusting the body within space because of proprioceptive feedback).

Control Before Capacity

Stability and Mobility in Unison

When proprioception and stability are working together in harmony, the body can achieve controlled functional movement. Mobility is the second half of control's source. Mobility is simply the freedom to move without restrictions. Sufficient mobility is mandatory to achieve the greatest amount of control possible. Stability and mobility must increase in unison. As you achieve new levels of mobility, you must be able to stabilize the range of motion, and as you improve stability, it allows you to support greater mobility. Remember, quality before quantity (Cook 2010). Once ample control is attained, the athletes can start enhancing their capacity. Capacity is the product of strength and metabolic capability. Strength is the aptitude to effectively execute stability and mobility at elevated levels and must be obtained prior to increasing metabolic ability to ensure proper movement as fatigue settles in and thus avoid injury.

Strength Comes Before Increasing Metabolic Ability

Metabolic ability is the capacity to sustain feats of strength over a sustained period. It is during metabolic training that athletes reach their potential. However, that potential cannot be reached or sustained without first adequately building the prior steps (stability, mobility, and strength). Metabolic function can be either aerobic or anaerobic depending on the demands of the sport, which lead to specific skills development. The training system being utilized should be sport specific the whole way through. When functional movement, mechanical integrity, and capacity are finally achieved, the athletes can begin fine-tuning their sport-specific skills. This is the time to train the specific demands of the physical feat(s) associated with their sports and when the athletes can achieve their true peak performance.

Most of what we as humans contribute to our success as a species arises from our astonishing minds. People are constantly in flux between creating novel ideas and identifying patterns. It is this combination of the unknown and known that allows us to spend energy engineering the world we live in while saving energy on familiar routines. However, our everyday movements are a feat of engineering that we as people tend to take shortcuts that cost us in the long run.

Survival Mechanism

PROformance Training Systems is designed to rebalance our body so that all the parts fire in sync, strengthen the individual parts and movement systems, and calibrate the human movement system toward athletic success.

The diagram below displays the chain of events allowing our basic survival instincts to take shortcuts and instigate injury during exercise and sport.

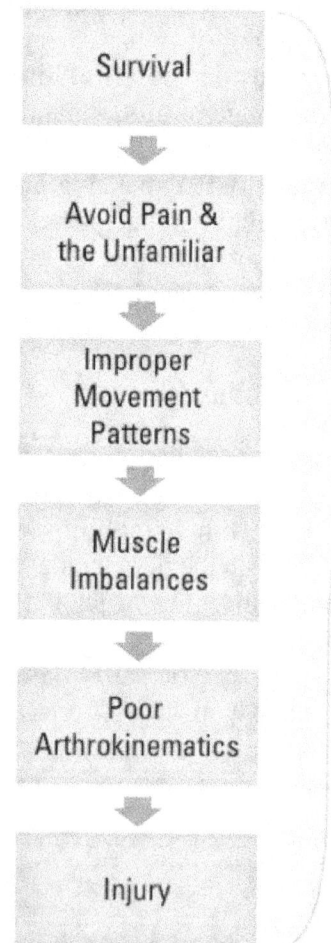

Humans by nature are creatures of extreme efficiency. As a result we take the path of least resistance. If we are weak in certain areas, improper movement patterns can occur. This leads to muscle imbalances and poor arthrokinematics (joint movement) that leads to injury. Our natural survival instincts tell us to avoid movements that cause pain or are unfamiliar even if they are natural. This leads to further pain and injury, creating an ongoing cycle.

We must re-educate our body to perform these basic movement patterns correctly in order to reduce injury and maximize performance. By relearning proper biomechanics from the beginning, we are allowing our bodies to perform in harmony with itself.

PROformance Training Systems

Functional Integrated Movements	Mechanical	Theme	Metabolic	Constant Evaluation & Systems Adaption
	Advanced Movement Systems & Max Power	Potential	**Specific Skills & Movements**	
	Maximize mechanical performance to allow optimal specific skills capability		Master movements and reactions to the demands of sport	
	Muscular Development III *Heavy Power*	Fortify	**Anaerobic Expansion**	
	Maximize connective tissue excitability and efficiency		Expand upon anaerobic capacity by implementing high intensity repetitions	
	Muscular Development II *Hypertrophy*		**Aerobic Capacity**	
	A hybrid between muscular development I & III		Improve the capacity at which oxygen can get to working muscles	
	Muscular Development I *Muscular Endurance*		**Threshold Development**	
	Increase the performance of metabolic pathways associated with repetitive muscle contraction		Establish resistance to fatigue at the ventilatory/ lactic threshold	
	Functional Stability & Neuromuscular Efficiency	Prepare	**Aerobic Elevation**	
	Improve motor control		Introduce aerobic elevation strategies to raise ventilatory threshold, increasing aerobic capacity	
	Basic Mobility & Corrective Strategies	Learn	**Metabolic Stimulation**	
	Work on any muscle imbalances & joint dysfunctions		Elevate heart rate in a novice & non-sports specific manner	

Mental Foundation & Support Structure
Motivation | Dedication | Resources

Mechanical	Learn	Prepare	Fortify	Potential
	Mobility *Sets* 2-3 *Reps* 12-15 *Rest* 60 s *Intensity* 1%-40%	Functional Stability *Sets* 3 *Reps* 12-15 *Rest* 30-45 s *Intensity* 50%-75%	Muscular Endurance *Sets* 3 *Reps* 12-15 *Rest* < 30 s *Intensity* 50%-75%	Max Power *Sets* 3-6 *Reps* 1-10 *Rest* 3-5 min *Intensity* 45% Or 10% Body Weight
	Corrective *Sets* 2-3 *Reps* 12-15 *Rest* 60 s *Intensity* 40%-60%	Neuromuscular Efficiency *Sets* 3 *Reps* 12-15 *Rest* 30-45 s *Intensity* 50%-75%	Hypertrophy *Sets* 3-4 *Reps* 4-12 *Rest* 45 s-2.5 min *Intensity* 75%-85%	Advanced Movement Systems *Sets* 3-6 *Reps* 1-10 *Rest* 3-5 min *Intensity* 100%
			Heavy Power *Sets* 4-6 *Reps* 1-4 *Rest* 3-5 min *Intensity* 85%-100%	
Metabolic	Learn	Prepare	Fortify	Potential
	Metabolic Stimulation *HR* 50%-60% *Reps* = Vary *Rest* = As needed	Aerobic Elevation *HR* 60%-80% *Reps* 1 *Rest* = Steady State	Threshold Development *HR* 80%-92% *Rest* 5:1 Ratio	Specific Movements *As Appropriate*
			Aerobic Capacity *HR* 92%-100% *Rest* 2:1-1:1 Ratio	Specific Skills *As Appropriate*
			Anaerobic Expansion *HR* 95%-100% *Rest* 1:3-1:5 Ratio	
Energy Refuel	**Muscle Fiber Activation**			
50% = 20-30 s 75% = 40 s 85%-90% = 60 s 100% = 3 min	Type I *Activation* 0% *Peak* 60% *Max* 80%	Type IIa *Activation* 60% *Peak* 85% *Peak* 100%	Type IIb *Activation* 90% *Peak* 100%+ *Max* 100%+	*These variables are for common use and can be adjusted.

The charts on the previous pages are PROformance Training Systems as a visual, and the following pages explain the system in more detail. As you will notice, I keep my lessons quick. I don't believe in ongoing chapters for the sake of writing a thick and impressive looking book. I understand what it is like to learn something, and there is no need to overcomplicate learning with unnecessary jargon. With that said, as the book progresses, you will discover some of the terminology can become dense with industry specific words, but this is a science book that at points references peer-reviewed literature and I want to deliver my lessons in a manner that stays true to the researcher's findings without it being overwhelming for an athlete who just wants to learn how to improve without too much thought into the science. Also, when speaking about the different parts of the body, if you do not have a background in anatomy and physiology it can become overwhelming, so I would recommend an overview of anatomy and physiology before reading any further. Remember, if you are just looking for straight forward answers, the "bold lines" and charts throughout the book will give you a quick summary of what I am explaining. Now, let's get into the fun stuff! What do the charts on the previous pages mean?

A system is an adapting method for performing a task. Whereas a program is fixed, a system changes with the situation. PTS consists of two domains: mechanical, which is composed of muscles, bones, tendons, ligaments, fascia, and so forth, and metabolic, consisting of energy systems, cardiovascular and cardiopulmonary development, and so forth. Both domains advance up the model in the following themes: learn, prepare, fortify, and potential (See diagram on previous page). The mission of the progression model is to advance human control and capacity to its upper limit by transcending and unifying the body mechanically and metabolically while considering the individual's mental commitment and social support. The main goal is to mold the athlete into his or her potential self.

Social and Mental Support is as Valuable to Performance as Physical Conditioning

The first theme is learn. This is where basic mechanical mobility is retaught to the individual, so they can use correct movement patterns during later development. We are all born with proper movement patterns, developing them as we age through trial and error. We lose the ability to perform these patterns correctly as we get older and lazier. This is a result of our body's natural desire to become more efficient. We take "movement shortcuts" to make motion more efficient, resulting in poor movement patterns and increased risk of injury. By undergoing corrective-exercise strategies and basic mobility drills, it reestablishes these movement patterns within the athlete, setting them up for success as they progress through the following themes.

As We Age, We Take Movement Shortcuts That Lead to Injury

Metabolic stimulation is also introduced during the learning theme. Here new and deconditioned athletes become reacquainted with an elevated heart rate in a fitness setting. This is accomplished by participating in non-sports-specific activities. It is important to think of the learning theme not as exercise but as priming the body for exercise in the following themes.

Preparing the body for advance development is the second theme. Mechanically, this takes place after efficient mobility is achieved but before muscular development training begins. Adequate mobility and sufficient stability must be in place before focusing on developing the musculature. If the body cannot move through a full range of motion and control those movements, the athlete is not prepared to undergo performance training. During this time, the athlete is performing functional stability and neuromuscular efficiency exercises to increase his or her bodily control, achieving acceptable levels of motion for the fortify stage. Metabolically, the body is being introduced to steady state cardio, elevating its aerobic capacity. By elevating aerobic capacity, it raises the anaerobic threshold; this makes aerobic elevation valuable for endurance and non-endurance sports. Fortification is the third theme of advancement.

Here muscular development strategies are introduced during mechanical training to improve the muscle fiber's energy systems and power development potential. Accomplishing this occurs over three stages. Muscular endurance is when the focus is on increasing the performance of metabolic pathways associated with repetitive muscle contractions. Muscular hypertrophy is a blend of muscular endurance and strength development, resulting in increased muscular size. The third stage, heavy power, focuses on maximizing connective tissue excitability and efficiency, for an increase in contraction speed and power.

On the metabolic side of the coin, threshold development, which is elevating your body's ventilatory threshold and lactate tolerance, is implemented through ventilatory and lactic threshold training. Threshold development training fortifies the body against fatigue while performing at the ventilatory/lactic threshold, allowing athletes to last longer at a higher-work rate than their competition. Once the threshold is fortified, aerobic capacity is established by improving the capacity at which oxygen can get to working muscles. High-intensity training done at VO_2max will help the muscles extract more oxygen from the bloodstream during high-intensity competition.

The final metabolic-fortification stage is anaerobic expansion, which expands upon anaerobic capacity by implementing high-intensity anaerobic repetitions. Anaerobic expansion is vital for reaching full athletic potential. Even a distance athlete undergoes anaerobic metabolism as acidosis accumulates in his or her legs. Furthermore, the adaptations that occur during anaerobic expansion activities are a necessary primer for the demands of the potential theme.

The final theme is potential, and it is here that athletes reach their athletic potential. Mechanically, this is accomplished through advanced movement systems consisting of power and maximum functional movement integration at full speed (training form drills). It is this stage of training that has the highest functional carryover to sport. Metabolically, this entails mastering movements and reactions to the demands of sport. These reactions can be movements or physiological demands. The goal of the potential theme is to unite the mechanical and metabolic components into one hybrid training method where the athlete can reach her potential. That said, it is important to note that just because one has reached a theme of the model, it does not mean they cannot regress back to a prior theme due to lack of training or poor training effort. HIIT training would be most applicable during this theme, harmonizing power, control, capacity, and skills.

Progress throughout PTS is determined through constant evaluation and systems adaptation to that evaluation. If the athlete does not pass the evaluation, then adapt the system to her needs. Moreover, since the individual is training her body for specific movements and physiological demands, it is vital that one treats the body as a singular system rather than a series of independent movements. The human movement system works as one unit; therefore, the model is meant to train the body using the most highly integrated functional movements applicable to each theme.

Mechanical Focuses on Strengthening Our Structure and Metabolic on Our Engine

	Mechanical	Theme	Metabolic	
Functional	Advanced Movement Systems *Power & Max Integrated Movement*	Potential	Anaerobic Expansion *VO$_2$ Max & Repetitions Maturity*	Constant
Integrated	Muscular Development *Endurance & Strength Enhancement*	Fortify	Threshold Capacity *Improve Work Capacity and Race Pace*	Evaluation
	Neuromuscular Efficiency *Improve Fire Order & Rate Efficiency*	Prepare	Aerobic Elevation *Raise Anaerobic Threshold*	&
Movements	Basic Mobility & Functional Stability *Re-educate, Proprioception, Balance*	Learn	Metabolic Stimulation *Elevate Heart Rate*	Systems Adaption

Additionally, once the goals of one theme are accomplished that theme is not forgotten as we progress up the hierarchy. The skills learned and abilities acquired are present in the integrated functional movements at the next level. All the traits and demands of the previous theme are present in the next one. This lessens the chance of reoccurrence of a mechanical limitation or metabolic detraining. Finally, but perhaps most important is the mental foundation and support structure of PROformance Training Systems; motivation, dedication, and resources.

Athletes need to be motivated toward their goal if they are going to be dedicated to the extent necessary to reach their true potential. Tremendous amounts of dedication in the form of commitment and consistency must be present if the athlete expects to adapt and progress up the themes. Constant mental sport coaching is a core element of a strong mental foundation. Moreover, adequate resources such as quality coaching, family and friend support, acceptable equipment, and ample time need to be available for athletes to undergo their training with the least amount of roadblocks. A strong mental foundation and solid support structure can consist of variable things depending on the athlete and sport. Therefore, it is vital to perform a consultation and follow-up consultation with the athlete on a regular basis, making certain that the needs of the foundation and structure have not changed and are still being met.

PROformance Training Systems is not the only method of progressing an individual toward excellence. However, based on my education and experience, it is one that I feel is highly justified and has been very successful for my athletes. Also, when possible perform the mechanical training prior to your metabolic training within a session. Mechanical training is more neurologically demanding and thus should be done first to ensure efficient control.

Perform Mechanical Training Before Metabolic Training

The Ten Most Common Fitness Questions Answered

Let's start with some quick questions and answers. I want to begin by clarifying the ten most commonly occurring fitness questions I hear on a regular basis. Below are what I think those questions are as well as my opinions on them.

1. How often should I exercise?

How often you should exercise depends on several factors. The major factors being goals, age, training age (how long you have been training), and medical history. The basic recommendations I give my clients can be found on the *PROformance Training Systems Exercise Recommendation Chart*. This chart is in the chapter "Why You're not Improving."

2. How do I get a flat stomach?

You can spend all day doing crunches at the gym trying to get a flat stomach, with the only result being frustration because nothing has changed. Having a flat stomach is more about body composition (the ratio of body fat to lean mass) than it is about the size of your abdominal muscles. If you want to have good abs, then increase your aerobic steady state (think jog through the park); high-intensity interval training, a.k.a. HIIT; and strength training to burn more fat. Strength training, especially lower-body strength training has been shown to increase testosterone and growth hormone post-exercise. Both hormones are essential for burning fat. Also, it has been said that weight loss is 80 percent what you eat and 20 percent exercise, so keep that in mind next time you think it's OK to have extra ice cream because you worked out. It's easier to not consume a calorie than burn one.

3. How do I get rid of these flabby arms?

When it comes to getting rid of flabby triceps on the posterior (back) side of your arm when waving, you cannot just isolate the muscle and wish the fat away. There is no such thing as spot reduction, otherwise known as isolating one area to burn fat at that location. However, if you eat a healthy diet aimed toward weight loss while also performing upper-body compound movements that include your triceps such as overhead shoulder press and chest press, you will lose weight and build up the muscles in your arms, so they look more defined. And females, although building strong muscles is essential for athletic excellence, if building big muscles is not your goal, don't worry as only about 1 percent of the female population have the genetic potential to be as big as a natural, competitive bodybuilder. Moreover, professional body building is its own discipline with unique goals, meaning if you are properly training for soccer or lacrosse, you will not look like a body builder. Males, you have roughly a 10 percent genetic potential to sculpt the build of a professional natural body builder.

4. Is breakfast really the most important meal of the day, and what's all this about several small meals throughout the day?

Breakfast is called that for a reason; you are "breaking fasting." With that said, fasting puts your body in a state of catabolism (breaking down muscle). Within thirty minutes of waking up, have a three-hundred- to five-hundred-calorie meal consisting of 30 percent protein. This will turn your body anabolic (build muscle and burn fat) again for roughly three to four hours. It is important to continue eating small meals throughout the day every three to four hours to remain anabolic. Two of your meals should be slightly larger than the rest. One of the two larger meals should be right before or after exercise.

5. Why are my muscles sore after a workout?

Your muscles are sore after a workout due to delayed-onset muscle soreness (DOMS). It's not during the workout that your muscles become bigger and stronger but after the workout when they are adapting to the stress they just underwent—remodeling, rebuilding, and hence hurting. DOMS can take twenty-four to seventy-two hours before you start to feel the aching and burning sensation that can accompany skeletal-muscle tissue remodeling, and it can last a couple of days after it begins. Your muscles will also hurt more when you are new to a certain exercise, deconditioned, or performing eccentric (emphasis on lengthening or "negative" movement) exercises.

6. Does muscle turn into fat?

No, a muscle turning into fat is a popular myth, but it holds no truth. What is happening when you think your muscles are turning into fat is as you become less active, your muscles atrophy (shrink). When muscles atrophy, your body's metabolism slows down, so you do not burn as many calories. At the same time, the excess calories you are consuming are stored as fat. It's not muscle turning into fat, rather muscle wasting and being replaced with fat.

7. What is the difference between free weights and weight machines?

Free weights are exercise tools such as dumbbells or barbells, whereas weight machines are more restrictive and used mostly for isolation exercises such as the pec deck or leg-extension machine. I personally believe free weights are the best way to functionally train people of all experience levels because they teach your body how to properly move through functional movement patterns by activating synergist muscles, enhancing firing rate, and ordering of muscle recruitment. This will produce better performance in athletes and boost metabolism in non-athletes by recruiting more muscle fibers. Free weights also enhance proprioception, improving bodily control. If I am working with an athlete who is too weak to handle the load of external weight, then I have them perform the movement with no weight until they are strong enough to handle free weights rather than load them up on a weight machine.

8. Why should I rest my muscles after a workout?

You should rest your muscles after a workout because it is after the workout that the adaptations occur causing you to become stronger and bigger. During the workout, you are causing micro tears to your myofibrils (contractile filament of a muscle) that during rest adapt to the new stress, so you are stronger and ready for your next workout or competition. Remember, your muscles need plenty of food to provide them with the nutrients they need to grow and water to stay hydrated.

9. What is my target heart rate?

There are a few formulas for estimating target heart rate. The most common one, the Karvonen formula, is as follows: Target Heart Rate = ([max HR − resting HR] × %Intensity) + resting HR. To find your max heart rate, it's 220 − your age.

Note: There can be some error when using this formula because people are so adaptable and varying to exercise.

10. What should I eat after a workout and why?

After you are done working out, you should eat a 3–4:1 ratio of carbohydrate to protein. This meal should be consumed within the first thirty minutes post-exercise while your body is still in an anabolic environment and should be mostly simple sugars and protein with a high-biological value (most similar to the form our body needs). This will speed up absorption and enhance the recovery process. The quicker we begin refueling empty glycogen (energy) stores and rebuilding broken down muscle tissue, the more we can get out of our next workout. It is also important to consume a 3–4:1 ratio of carbohydrates to protein before a workout because it takes roughly sixty to ninety minutes for the food to digest and enter the bloodstream. By having a small meal before your workout, it allows the nutrients to be prepared for absorption when your workout is finished. If you are in dietary distress from this small meal, adjust accordingly. Remember, it's not a single food's chemical composition that matters, rather the composition of the entire meal. Keep this in mind when planning your diet.

Exercise places a lot of stress on the body. When we begin exercising, we are taking it from a comfortable state of rest to an all-out frenzy. This task can be a shock to our system if we are not prepared for it. Therefore, it is important to perform a dynamic warm-up prior to exercise. When we warm up, we are preparing ourselves for exercise in multiple ways. For starters, we are enhancing vasodilatation in our arteries and veins, which allows them to pump more blood to our muscles and clear by-products quicker, allowing more energy to be consumed by our muscles during physical activity.

This process also helps warm up our muscles, allowing oxygen carried in the blood to detach from hemoglobin and be used by muscles. If our muscles are not warmed up properly, the oxygen does not want to detach from the hemoglobin. In other words, if we go straight into exercise without warming up, our arteries will deliver less oxygen to our muscles, and the oxygen that is delivered will not want to detach from the hemoglobin and enter our muscles, resulting in a lower volume of oxygen available for use by your muscles. Additionally, as our bodies heat up, the capillaries interacting with our working muscles dilate allowing more oxygen-rich blood and by-products to enter and exit our muscles with greater ease.

Moving away from the importance of warming-up with respects to blood flow is the benefit our nervous system receives. As our nervous system heats up, the electrical impulses are sent with more efficiency to the working muscles from our central and peripheral nervous system (brain and spinal cord). As a result, our reaction time is improved, and enhanced reaction time means enhanced performance.

Finally, when our body is warmer, we use our energy more efficiently. The fat we release into our bloodstream during exercise can be utilized much better when our muscles are warm than when they are cold. Cold muscles will not use as many fatty acids as warm muscles. Therefore, when our muscles are cold and not warmed up properly, the fatty acids released into our bloodstream end up in unwanted places such as our arteries.

Looking back at all this, it is obvious that warming up has greater benefits to it than simply avoiding pulling a muscle. Now that we know our performance is significantly enhanced when we warm up first, we appreciate how making time for a proper warm-up is key to excellence. With that said, give yourself ten to twenty minutes prior to engaging in intense activity to slowly bring your body up to speed by performing a light-to-moderate metabolic training followed by mobility drills and ending with sport-specific drills.

Warm-Up for 10-20 Min Prior to Intense Physical Activity

Static stretching is the most common muscle-lengthening technique used prior to exercise as part of a warm-up. It is believed to improve range of motion (ROM) as well as inhibit overactive neuromyofacial tissue, resulting in increased performance. Recent interest in stretching's effects on athletic performance have elicited mixed reviews from athletes and coaches. Recent articles detail stretching's place in exercise as potentially helpful, but note that static stretching decreases power and should be used in combination with other modalities such as practice drills and low-intensity dynamic exercises if stretching is necessary at all (McHugh and Cosgrave 2010). While others found the power-diminishing effects of stretching to diminish when performed prior to high-intensity sport-specific skills based activity (Taylor et al. 2009), these findings suggest stretching does have its place in exercise when used in conjunction with a proper warm-up.

Until recently, scientists did not fully understand how static stretching works. However, within recent years new research has been developed regarding static stretching and its effects on the mechanisms involved. Research shows pre-exercise stretching increases the activation of Golgi tendon organs (GTO), which decrease motor-neuron excitability and muscle-spindle excitability. This results in decreased cross-bridge formation and consequently a decrease in performance. What does this all mean in English? When your muscles are tight (overactive), there are motor neurons and muscles spindles (sensory receptors in muscle cells that detect elongation of the muscle) that are activating the things that contract and come together (cross bridges). Now when we are not exercising, these motor neurons and muscles spindles are supposed to turn off. If they are not, it can lead to muscle imbalances and possible dysfunctional movement patterns. So these things called GTOs are supposed to come along and turn off the things that cause the stretch (motor neurons and muscle spindles). GTOs are part of the reason why you lose tension during an exercise, they come in as a safety mechanism to stop you before you hurt yourself. The GTOs are activated by either pressure or stretching the overactive area. The stretch should last for twenty to thirty seconds (sixty seconds for individuals over fifty years) and can be repeated for up to four times.

Stretching and Pressure Relieve Tight Muscles

The question of what to do with respect to stretching in an exercise program can finally be answered. According to McHugh et al. (2010), stretching should not be performed in isolation and is best utilized with other aspects of a pre-participation warm-up. Taylor et al. (2009) found similar findings when attempting to determine if the inhibiting effects static stretching produce on performance can be reversed with high-intensity skill-based warm ups. Taylor and colleagues determined that in fact stretching combined with other warm-up drills restore the difference lost from stretching alone.

Since static stretching decreases performance, is stretching prior to exercise worth it? This one is still up in the air for the most part. However, most scientists agree acute stretching directly prior to a workout is useless unless it is part of a corrective-exercise regimen put in place to inhibit overactive tissue. But, chronic stretching daily has been shown to increase ROM.

To understand how static stretching works, let's look at its deeper impact on performance. Remember how stretching decreases cross-bridge formation (the contractile filaments sliding together). Well, it's that cross-bridge formation that is giving you your strength. The more cross bridges a muscle has, the higher your strength and power output (read "How

Muscle Is Made"). Studies show there is a decrease in strength and power after static stretching. Also, this decrease will negatively impact all power and strength related activities for ten to sixty minutes post-stretch. Therefore, it is highly advisable to avoid static stretching prior to strength or power-related training sessions.

It is also worth noting that most people do not stretch properly, stretching an overactive muscle can accidently overstretch the adjacent muscles that do not require stretching because the adjacent muscles are healthy and thus stretch whereas the overactive muscle is over-contracting and thus not willing to stretch. This can cause an unintentional lengthening of a healthy muscle, leading to further dysfunction. For this reason, I recommend myofascial release (applying pressure) to overactive muscles prior to stretching.

Walking away from this, remember to perform a dynamic warm-up prior to your workout and a static stretch afterward as part of your daily routine. Do not perform static stretching prior to strength or power-related activities, rather perform a full dynamic warm-up and save static stretching for after. The only time you would stretch before a workout is when there is known tight connective tissue, and even then, use pressure therapy on the muscle prior to stretching.

Perform a Dynamic Warm-Up Before Exercise and Static Stretching After Exercise

Body composition is a measurement of the human body concerned with fat, muscle, bone, and water density. Measurements of body composition give insight into an individual's health and physical fitness as an individual and compared to his or her peers.

Body composition can be measured using numerous methods. The most popular of these methods are skinfold caliper test, hydrostatic weighing, bioelectrical impedance analysis (BIA), dual-energy x-ray absorptiometry (DEXA), whole-body air displacement plethysmography (ADP), magnetic resonance imaging (MRI), and computed tomography (CT). This chapter is motivated by three research questions: (1) Can body composition statistics bring valuable information and predictions concerning mortality, cardiovascular health, and risk of periodontitis? (2) What is the accuracy of these leading body-composition measurement methods? (3) Does ergogenic supplementation effectively alter body composition?

The value of measuring body composition

Previous research concerning body composition and mortality indicates that body mass index (BMI) and loss of skeletal-muscle mass is positively correlated with all-cause mortality, heart failure, periodontitis, and coronary artery disease in adults (Goodpaster et al. 2006; Loehr et al. 2009; Orpana et al. 2010; Szulc et al. 2010; Romero-Corral et al. 2006; Salekzamani et al. 2011). These findings reveal a positive correlation between a variety of serious health concerns with body composition. This insight can act as an early warning sign for these health conditions, since body composition has been shown in previous research to decrease naturally as people age (Borkan et al. 1983).

High BMI is Positively Correlated with All-Cause Mortality

It is of importance for people to begin monitoring and developing a healthy body composition at an early age. Knowing this, two questions need to be asked. First, what are the safest and most effective methods of reaching healthy BMI and skeletal-muscle-mass percentages. Second, just how accurate are these body-composition measurement methods?

Central to the science of body-composition measurement is the methods used to measure body composition as well as accuracy of those methods. A considerable amount of literature has been published on the accuracy of body-composition measurements. Drawing on Moon et al.'s (2009b) literature, Jackson et al.'s sum of three skinfold equations is an acceptable method of measuring fat-percentage values in Division I female athletes. However, comparative studies found that skinfold measurements, dual-energy x-ray absorptiometry, and bioelectrical impedance analysis are not accurate measures of measuring body composition (LaForgia et al. 2009; Minderico et al. 2008; Santos et al. 2010; Silva et al. 2009). Specifically compared to three-, four-, five-, and six-compartment body-composition models (Moon et al. 2009; Wang et al. 1998; Withers et al. 1998), this knowledge of body-composition measurement accuracy allows medical practitioners to have a better understanding of the accuracy of their measurements and what they can safely assume from those findings given the measurement device being used.

Ergogenic supplementation can have benefits for underweight, overweight, and obese people considered at high health risk. Research by Kreider et al. (1998) and Mårin et al. (1992) show that supplementation with ergogenic aids such as creatine, taurine, glucose, electrolytes, and testosterone can aid in altering body composition by bringing body composition to healthy benchmarks.

Ergogenic Supplementation is Proven to Aid in Altering Body Composition

Findings from the research on body composition and mortality illustrate how a reduction in appendicular skeletal muscle mass can lead to mortality in older men (Szulc et al. 2010). Furthermore, Goodpaster and colleagues (2006) show that the impact of aging on loss of skeletal-muscle strength in older adults is aging associated and is not prevented by maintaining muscle mass. Strength loss in older adults is apparent from their findings showing lean mass as independent from strength decline.

Strong evidence of body mass index having an impact on mortality was made clear from Orpana (2010) analysis of the 1994/1995 National Population Health Survey (Canada). Orphan and colleagues suggest underweight and obesity are both at higher risk for mortality. Whereas overweight had a significantly decreased risk of death, Romero-Corral et al. (2006) found similar results suggesting overweight and mildly obese individuals show better outcomes of mortality than normal and low-body-mass-index individuals. Furthermore, studies by Loehr and colleagues (2009) found obesity and overweight individuals were associated with heart failure, while a study by Salekzamnani et al. (2011) found a positive correlation between severe forms of periodontal disease in males and their body composition. These results show poor body composition negatively impacts quality of life on a multitude of levels.

Quality of Life Decreases as Body Composition Increases to Unhealthy Levels

Accuracy

Contrary to our expectations, when comparing methods of accurately measuring body composition, many of the methods were proven inaccurate (LaForgia et al. 2009; Minderico et al. 2008; Santos et al. 2010; Silva et al. 2009; Wang et al. 1998). Lafarge and colleagues (2009) showed dual-energy x-ray absorptiometry loses accuracy when estimating obese men and women because of tissue thickness. Similar findings were observed implying skinfold as well as dual-energy x-ray absorptiometry are not accurate measures of body composition in a range of people from overweight and obese women (Minderico et al. 2008) to elite Judo athletes (Silva et al. 2009; Santos et al. 2010).

The key limitation of the above research is lack of accurate body composition measurement. However, most of the previous studies did not consider three-, four-, five-, and six-compartment models used in clinical settings to search for body-composition measurement accuracy. Results show these methods are valid for estimating percent body fat in female college athletes (Moon et al. 2009a, 2009b). The difference in accuracy between body-composition measurement methods can foreshadow life or death according to the above research on mortality and body composition.

Body Composition Measurement Devices are Still Prone to Error

Ergogenic supplementation

Findings on ergogenic aid supplementation showed testosterone boosting as well as performance enhancing substances such as testosterone, creatine, or creatine with taurine, glucose, and electrolytes have a profound impact on lean mass. Results showed supplementation with these substances increased lean mass beyond that of daily activities or exercise without ergogenic aids (Kreider et al. 1998; Mårin et al. 1992).

Ergogenic Aids Were Shown to Increase Lean Mass

Overall

Discussing the above findings, it was the main purpose of this chapter to draw attention to a growing body of research on body composition over the past decades due to advances in science and technology allowing medical and health practitioners to improve upon previous body-composition models. However, many of the topics discussed above are comparing aged measurement techniques such as caliper test with new technologies such as dual-energy x-ray absorptiometry. Differences in accuracy and available statistics between such methods are bound to exist. However, aging-measurement models are still of interest for less serious scenarios where accuracy is not essential or dangerous to the outcome; for example, if there are slight inaccuracies such as personal trainers using skinfold calipers to measure body composition in a fitness club setting with an apparently healthy client, these methods may be more common in places such as fitness clubs due to financial restrictions. Although the measurement may not be perfect, it can give the fitness professionals the opportunity to suggest to their client that they go for a more accurate medical examination.

Moreover, these methods of measuring body composition were developed to provide early warning to health risk such as heart failure, mortality, and more recently periodontitis (inflammation of the tissue surrounding the teeth). Body composition measurement tools are essential for monitoring progress of an overweight or obese individual's journey back to a healthy weight range. By encouraging overweight and obese people to have their body composition measured on a weekly or monthly basis, it may give them enough positive feedback and motivate them to begin or continue losing weight.

Body Composition is an Accurate Indicator of Health Risk

Furthermore, ergogenic-aid supplementation has a critical place in helping people who are either incapable of improving their body composition on their own due to sickness, age, or injury or are looking to improve body composition for athletic prosperity.

From the reviewed research, it is possible to conclude that body composition brings valuable information and predictions concerning mortality, cardiovascular health, and periodontal status. Attention was also given to the accuracy of the leading body-composition measurement methods. Results revealed body-composition measurement methods vary drastically and such knowledge should be considered when performing body-composition measurements. The findings suggest monitoring body composition could also be useful for catching early warning signs of other health concerns. The above studies only focus on a few health issues. However, there are numerous other health issues that can be avoided, stopped, or slowed down with enough early detection and warning. Understanding an individual's body composition allows them to know where his or her health is going (improving, stable, or declining) as well as how to change that prediction through diet and exercise intervention with ergogenic aids when appropriate. Further research on body composition is desirable to extend the fields knowledge of health implications associated with varying body-composition types.

Strength and conditioning are subcategories of exercise physiology pertaining specifically to increasing the mechanical and metabolic capacity of athletes. Strength and conditioning coaches utilize exercise prescription to manipulate training variables such as exercise type, frequency, intensity, duration, and rest to improve range of motion, stability, neuromuscular efficiency, aerobic and muscular endurance, hypertrophy, strength, aerobic capacity, and power. Exercise prescription is selected based upon the demands of the sport and individual needs of the athlete. Every athlete including those involved in the same position for a given sport will need a slightly different training protocol based upon his or her training history, age, gender, skill, desire, and medical history.

The following chapter examines three main areas. First research concerning concurrent strength and endurance training protocols will be investigated to determine if the two disciplines work synergistically or interfere with one another. Next, we will examine whether single or multiple sets produce better results, then we will look into what time of day is best for strength training. Dwelling upon whether morning or afternoon strength training produces the best results.

Several articles reported concurrent resistance- and endurance-training regimes do not impede one and other as previously thought but rather suggest synergy between the two training modalities. These findings were found to be true for general exercise among apparently healthy males (Shaw, Shaw, and Brown, 2009). Integrated concurrent exercise (a blend of strength and endurance training during a single session) is a better training method compared with linear concurrent exercise (a complete strength session followed by a complete endurance session) among female college athletes (Davis et al. 2008).

Concurrent Training is More Effective Than Linear Training

Comparable findings were found to be true for males and females attempting to improve running economy by combining it with maximal strength training (Støren et al. 2008). Støren and colleagues learned time to exhaustion increased after eight weeks of maximal strength training in conjunction with participants' normal running regimen. Similar research by Sunde and Helgerud (2010) discovered maximal strength training over an eight-week period also enhances cycling economy in competitive cyclist.

Although differences in results were apparent due to different methods and procedures of measuring concurrent resistance and endurance training among respective participants, the general census that a combination of strength and endurance training produces beneficial results for general population as well as endurance athletes appears true. For more on this topic, I recommend reading my other book, *PR Pace: Strength & Performance Training for Distance Runners.*

Two conflicting articles regarding whether multiple sets of resistance training offer any benefit over single set of resistance training have found contradictory findings. Krieger (2009) results found two to three sets to be better for strength training than a single set by 46 percent, but no significant difference between one set and four to six sets or two to three sets and four to six sets. Whereas research conducted by Carpinelli and Otto found no significant difference in the increase in strength or hypertrophy when comparing single versus multiple sets. These results show conflicting findings that leave room for further research; however, Carpinelli and Otto (1998) mention there are design limitations to the studies they examined, therefore do not completely neglect multiple set training. Moreover, rest intervals influence sets in numerous ways, as you will learn later in this book.

In One Study, 2-3 Sets Was 46% Better for Strength Training Than a Single Set

After a thorough examination of the relationship between strength and endurance training on a range of disciplines for both men and women, it appears that for periods lasting between eight and sixteen weeks a combination of strength training integrated with endurance training or performed separately as a supplement to their normal endurance training improve strength as well as aerobic economy (running and cycling) (Shaw et al. 2009; Davis et al. 2008; Stören et al. 2008, and Sunde et al. 2010).

An examination of the best time of day to strength train for men brought about consistent findings across the board from three similar studies. Sedliak et al. (2009) found after ten weeks of strength training that there was no significant difference in hypertrophy of quadriceps femoris muscle size regardless of time-of-day training. Sedliak et al. (2007) found similar results during their examination on time-of-day training on hormone concentrations and isometric strength in men. After ten weeks, the twenty- to forty-five-year-olds showed a reduction in morning cortisol levels compared to afternoon cortisol levels but summed it up to decreased masking effects of anticipatory psychological stress taking place before morning testing. Testosterone levels were found to be the same and maximal isometric strength was lower in the morning than the afternoon. A final study by Sedliak and colleagues (2008) showed mixed results for their examination of EMG activity during the morning compared with the afternoon. Although some results showed a significant difference in peak torque between morning and afternoon training, results varied between individuals.

The literature at hand unleashes multiple findings to the world of strength and conditioning. The first and foremost diminishes the myth that strength training produces negative consequences among endurance athletes. The greatest strength behind the articles related to combining strength and endurance training is that the research design and sampling is multigender and multisport. By studying males and females from general fitness to running and cycling, it shows less bias than a group of articles focusing on a specific demographic.

Strength Training Does Not Hinder Endurance Athletes

Second is whether single set or multiple sets are best for strength training. This topic reveals mixed findings; however, leaning toward multiple sets does seem to be more beneficial than single-set training at this point. If all other variables are considered a wash between the two training protocols, multiple sets can be viewed as additional time practicing the movement and building up to an effective training intensity/load versus only performing the movement for one set. This also provides a positive endocrine response discussed in a later chapter, "Hormonal Responses to Exercise, Nutrition, Age, and Gender."

Multiple Sets Deliver Compound Benefits

Finally, the best time of day to strength train was examined and found to be nearly irrelevant with only a single study suggesting possible benefits in morning strength training over afternoon strength training. These findings are a sign of relief for individuals feeling confined by their work/exercise schedule and believe they are limited by the time of day they are forced to exercise. My personal preference concerning when to exercise is to start your day right by getting in a workout. This way, regardless of how the rest of your day goes, you at least accomplished one good thing.

Exercise When Time Allows, Rather than Struggling for a Specific Time of Day

In closing, strength and conditioning encompass an expansive compendium of training methods based on the goals of the individual (power, strength, endurance, flexibility, etc.) as well as methods to manipulate those modalities such as frequency, duration, intensity, and rest. By gaining a better understanding of how these training methods interact with each other and are responded to by the body, it gives athletes and coaches an advantage, allowing them to better systematically devise a plan for the athlete to improve. The more science reveals about how the body responds to exercise, the further sport can push into the unknown. Athlete performance is only as good as the training.

How Long Should Each Theme Last?

PROformance Training Systems Theme Duration Breakdown				
Phase	**Metabolic**	**Mechanical**	**Duration (Weeks)**	**Resistance Phase Breakdown**
Learn	Aerobic Pace	Corrective	8–16	1/3
		Stability		
	Long and Slow Distance	Endurance		
Prepare	Long Intervals	Hypertrophy	4–6	1/2
	Tempo and Race Pace	Strength		
Fortify	VO$_2$Max	Explosive Power	2–4	1
	Short Repetition			
Potential	Aerobic	Plyometrics/ Corrective	1–3	Varies

This matrix is One Way an Athlete Could Progress Through a Macrocycle Following PTS

Training theory or periodization is simply a method of systematically scheduling and planning your training cycle. It encompasses cycles altering the intensity and volume of training so you can peak at the perfect time and reach your full potential (see the chart on the previous page). The basic set up behind training theory is there are three types of cycles. A macrocycle is the total training period; this typically lasts one year for most athletes. A mesocycle is typically four to six weeks long, and a microcycle commonly lasts between seven and ten days. These cycles are happening at the same time one within the other. This is how training theory works, strategically moving through small phases of training making up a bigger phase of training. The point of training is to adapt and get better, is it not? And athletes get better by adding new stimulus to their body. Their body will take this unknown stimulus and adapt to it becoming stronger and faster. Work is put in place to activate the adaptation stage, but once the work is complete, we allow for the adaptation to take place. This occurs during the rest/recovery phase. Our body adapts during the rest/recovery phase. This is when we get better, not during the work itself. To understand this better, picture a section of rolling hills from a side view. Each hill goes up and then back down. However, when they go down, they are not going as far down as the previous hill, but they go slightly higher on the next hill. This is how the adaptation process works. We go up and then down a little to recover, and because we recovered and got better, we can go even higher the next time.

Recovery Time is Essential for Progress

Let's take this one more step. We understand we have cycles (macro, meso, and micro), and the purpose of these cycles is to adapt to a stimulus to improve. But how do we properly add a training stimulus without over killing it or not adding enough? That is where intensity and volume come into play. Intensity is how hard we are training, and volume is how much we are training. Picture two water towers side by side sharing the same water supply. There is only enough water for one tower to be full at a time. Therefore, they should share the water evenly. Some days tower A will get more water than tower B, and other days tower B will have more water than tower A. But they will never both be full at the same time. This is how the intensity-to-volume relationship works. As one goes up, the other must go down to compensate. You can never have them both up for too long or else the athlete will burn out.

How you decide to break up the intensity-to-volume ratio depends on the phase in the cycle. Every micro, meso, and macro cycle will go from levels of high volume, low intensity to levels of high intensity, low volume depending on the training objective. The key is understanding the elements of that objective and purpose so you can design your training cycle effectively.

Note: In this chapter, I am referring to heavy-resistance loads or sprint repetitions as high intensity, although high volume running, cycling, swimming, hiking, and so on are also a form of high-intensity training.

Micro = Days; Meso = Weeks; Macro = Years

Exercise and DNA

Every day millions of people exercise, some for aesthetics and some for health. But just how big of a difference is exercise making on our body's structure on a molecular level? Does exercise change our DNA? Are these changes permanent? Will they be passed down to my children? How much exercise is necessary to bring about these changes? Insight brought to light by discoveries with the human genome project have given us answers to these questions regarding our athletic fate and if we can change it.

Does exercise change our DNA? No, exercise does not change the DNA code; however, the way the code is read is changed. DNA is decorated with chemical tags determining the way DNA is read. Exercise has been found to add or take away these chemical tags, changing the way DNA is read. When the code is read differently, it changes the way it interacts with other proteins. These new interactions resulting from exercise promote growth and metabolism. This is accomplished by improving the way muscles store and utilize sugar and fats as energy sources.

Are these changes permanent? After a twenty-minute bout of very strenuous exercise, the alterations were apparent that promote growth and metabolism; however, after exercise ceased, these changes disappeared. Despite this, during the recovery period, there was eminence of the growth and metabolism changes even without the DNA change. Whether these changes stay for the long term or are passed down to your offspring was not determined.

What is the necessary amount of exercise to elicit these changes? After comparing exercise at 40 percent and 80 percent max capacity, it was determined that exercising for thirty-five minutes at high intensity is adequate activating the changes in DNA that support sugar and fat metabolism after exercise.

20 min very Strenuous/35 Min High Intensity = Muscle Growth, Sugar and Fat Metabolism

It's a question as old as athletics itself. What is the underlying factor in excelling in sports? Is it genetics or hard work? We all know that there are certain limitations to our body that allow us to enhance our performance to a certain point where we reach the "genetic ceiling," but that level is usually lowered by a person's own willingness to perform far before he reaches his true potential.

I'm not saying all people are lazy; what I am saying is most of us have much more to give as athletes than we do. Numerous studies have shown that world class athletes don't simply have better genetics than the average person, but they work longer and harder. Research has shown that there is an underlying factor commonly referred to as the "motivation gene" driving people toward excellence. It is this gene and not superior muscle fiber type, lactate threshold, or any other athletic factor that separates the common person from the elite. It is their pursuit of excellence that makes them successful.

There is a Motivation Gene That is a Large Contributor to Excellence

Perhaps the elite have more drive and put in more time training than we do. Obvious statement I know, but the elite were not always the elite, were they? They all started as people just like you and I with a dream of achieving big things. The difference is their competitive spirit that leads them toward that dream. Yes, there is a certain level of athletic ability the elite possess, but there is a surprising amount of people out there with athletic talent who choose not to build upon it. One study claimed that there is one child in every classroom with the physical genetic capacity to be an Olympian, but they lack the will to get there.

Olympic Potential is More Common Than You May Think

It's the drive in an individual that allows her to shape her path and choose her destiny. All of us, whatever our talent level, can excel in sport; we must want to do so. The key is to understand what it takes to get to where we want to be then act upon it. The only thing stopping any one of us from being excellent is our own belief that we are not.

Although elites have biomechanical, physiological, and metabolic advantages, it's not some genetically superior gift that makes them great but rather the competitive engineering that occurs in their body when they want something badly and are willing to make sacrifices for it. If it were purely their physical traits that make elite athletes excellent, then more of their children would be high level athletes. How many professional athlete's children go pro? Not many, because they lack the drive their parents possess. We all know the sacrifices it entitles. The question is, are we willing to make those sacrifices for the thrill, pleasure, and fulfillment of excellence in sport?

Endocrinology is the study of the endocrine system, which is a collection of secretion glands responsible for transporting hormones to distant organs influencing functions and behaviors. As a subdiscipline of biology, endocrinology is concerned with functions of living organisms ranging from sleep and stress to movement and respiration (Nelson 2005).

The endocrine system is composed of several glands secreting hormones directly into the blood rather than into a duct system. In some cases, an organ may have multiple hormones acting upon it, while other instances may have a single hormone that has a variety of effects on multiple organs. Hormones can be further divided into three distinct classes depending on their chemical composition amines, peptides and proteins, and steroids (Ojeda and Griffin 2000).

The following chapter examines the endocrine system's response to exercise and sports under a variety of conditions beginning with exercise and sports hormonal response to varying training intensities, durations, frequency, and rest interval as well as nutritional intervention and its impact on performance. Progressing to endocrine responses in elderly men because of participation in exercise and supplementation. Finally ending with the hormonal influences on exercise during women's menstrual cycle.

Beginning with *The Physiology of Growth Hormone and Sport* (2009), it has been long known growth hormone (GH)/insulin-like growth factor-I (IGF-I) has short- and long-term metabolic effects, improving traits important to exercise including maximal oxygen uptake (VO_2max) and ventilatory threshold (VeT). Exercise has been shown to be a potent stimulus to GH release, and there is evidence that an acute increase in GH is important in regulating substrate metabolism post-exercise. Furthermore, regular exercise increases twenty-four-hour GH secretion rates, promoting physiological changes induced by training. An effective method of measuring these changes is studying GH replacement in GH-deficient adults and examining the long-term implications. Widdowson, Healy, Sunken, and Gibney (2009) found convincing evidence that GH replacement increases exercise capacity. Performance increases are thought to be due to increased fatty-acid availability with glycogen sparing, increased muscle strength, improved body composition, and improved thermoregulation. Moreover, administration of supraphysiologic doses of GH to athletes was shown to increase fatty-acid availability and reduce oxidative-protein loss specifically during exercise as well as increase lean body mass.

Widdowson et al. noted it is not known whether these effects translate to improved athletic performance, even though GH abuse is known in sports. These findings support reason for further research on natural methods of raising GH by manipulating exercise intensity, duration, frequency, and rest. If more effective methods of naturally increasing GH can be found, then athletes may be persuaded to reduce supplemental GH intake.

GH Levels Increase with Compound Lower-body Strength Training

Doping

Another study by Gibney, Healy, and Sönksen (2007) also looks at adult GH deficiency and the effects of GH-replacement therapy to learn more about growth hormone/insulin-like growth factor-I in exercise and sport. By learning measures of exercise performance such as maximal oxygen uptake and ventilatory threshold are impaired in adult GH deficiency and improved by GH replacement along with improved glycogen sparing, increased muscle strength, improved body composition, and improved thermoregulation, which are also traits of athletic performance. There is reason to believe that supraphysiological doses of GH to athletes improve physical performance although there is lack of evidence proving this. Moreover, it has been known that athletes abuse GH, and governing bodies are implementing tests to detect GH abuse. Both Widdowson et al. and Gibney et al. findings can help sport-medicine professionals to properly treat injured athletes with low GH levels by supplementing them with supervised medical GH treatment. Medically supervised GH treatment can help bring injured athletes back to healthy activity quicker during rehabilitation.

Being that GH abuse in sports is prevalent, athletes are turning to doping with insulin-like growth factor-I (IGF-I) since its detection methods are still not as well established as GH or testosterone. Guha, Sönksen, and Holt (2009) reveal current knowledge and prospects for detection of IGF-I. IGF-I is considered a substitute in athletics for GH since IGF-I's availability has increased from commercial preparations for use in disorders of growth, which makes its availability on the black market easier, and it mediates many of the anabolic actions of GH. IGF-I stimulates muscle protein synthesis, promotes glycogen storage, and enhances lipolysis. Long-term adverse effects of IGF-I administration are currently unknown but are thought to be like those of GH. Athletic governing bodies have already begun research into the detection of IGF-I abuse on the measurement of markers of GH action. There appears to be a cat and mouse game with hormone abusing athletes and scientist. As soon as a detection method is created for one performance-enhancing hormone, another hormone is abused in its place. This cat and mouse game brings up an ethical question, is it better to ban performance-enhancing substances or would it be better to develop a safe performance-enhancement substance that is provided and monitored by qualified medical staff? This ethical question is beyond our current scope but is worth further research at a later time.

How does this impact bodybuilders?

Concerning anabolic and catabolic hormones effect during specific physical training protocols, Mäestu, Eliakim, Jarimäe, Valter, and Jürimäe (2010) investigate simultaneous effects of energy balance, caloric intake, and the hormonal anabolic-catabolic balance in bodybuilders prior to competition. Fourteen male bodybuilders underwent an energy-restricted period to reduce body fat for eleven weeks. The subjects were divided into two groups. The energy-restricted group (ERG) (n = 7), who were preparing for a competition, and the control group (CG) (n = 7), who continued to train regularly and did not change their dietary or training regimen. Participants were tested on three different occasions prior to competition for diet, body composition, and fasting hormonal assessment at eleven weeks (T1), five weeks (T2), and three days (T3).

Result showed a significant decrease of three anabolic pathways (insulin-like growth factor, insulin, and testosterone) from severe energy restriction to extremely low body-energy reserves that took place during the experiment regardless of high-protein intake. Mäestu et al. suggest monitoring of insulin and insulin-like growth factor concentrations to prevent losses in muscle mass during energy-restricted periods. Other nutritional precautions may be needed to maintain an anabolic state while in energy-restricted conditions. This study could be taken a step further to determine if increasing sleep would promote a greater anabolic state in the ERG group. Studies show GH-release peaks during sleep (Sonntag et al. 1982, 35–39). This GH increase by increasing sleep may increase anabolism enough to offset the decline in anabolic pathways from a severe energy restricted diet.

Adding Sleep Increases GH Levels, Potentially Offsetting the Effects of a Poor Diet

Whereas the research of Mäestu et al. manipulated nutritional factors to determine their influence on the endocrine system, "Hormonal Responses to Different Resistance Exercise Schemes of Similar Total Volume" (2009) assessed the effect of different resistance-exercise scheme (RES) designs of similar total load lifted on the responses of testosterone, cortisol, and creatine kinase (CK). The participants were twenty-seven healthy males performing varying volumes (repetitions × sets × load) on the bench press. Participants performed one of four volume schemes described by the One-repetition maximum (1RM) load: four sets of maximum repetitions at 50 percent 1RM, five sets of maximum repetitions at 75 percent 1RM, ten sets of maximum repetitions at 90 percent 1RM, or eight sets of maximum repetitions at 110 percent 1RM. Blood samples collected pre- and post-exercise at one and twenty-four hours (post) were analyzed for total and free testosterone, total cortisol, and CK. Little change was shown among testosterone and cortisol levels between different RES. Most likely because of the relatively low volume lifted and/or the small muscle mass activated by the bench press exercise. The 75 percent 1RM RES showed the greatest increase of cortisol and CK elevation, thereby suggesting an optimal blend of resistance and volume.

Five Sets of 75% 1RM Increases Anabolic Response During Bench Press

The results of Uchida, Crewther, Ugrinowitsch, Bacurau, Moriscot, and Aoki's (2009) study confirm previous recommendations regarding the prescription of resistance exercise and the importance of total volume as a stimulus for activating the endocrine system and achieving long-term adaptions. This study could be taken a step further and reproduced using the squat or conventional deadlift, which encompasses significantly more skeletal-muscle mass and may produce different results from the small muscle mass involved with the bench press.

Another study focusing on resistance training's effects on the endocrine system was performed by Willoughby and Taylor (2004) and looks to learn if sequential resistance exercise bouts influences serum testosterone (TST), sex hormone-binding globulin (SHBG) and free androgen index (FAI), skeletal muscle AR mRNA and protein expression, and myofibril protein content. Participants were eighteen untrained males randomly assigned to either a resistance-training [(RST (N = 9)] or control group [CON (N = 9)]. The RST performed three bouts of lower-body resistance exercises, each separated by forty-eight hours. Each exercise bout consisted of three sets of eight to ten repetitions at 75–80 percent one-repetition maximum using the squat, leg press, and leg extension exercise, respectively. Whereas the CON group performed no resistance training.

Three Sets at 75-80% 1RM Increases Anabolic Response During Leg Exercises

Data was collected through muscle biopsies that were performed immediately before the first exercise bout and forty-eight hours after each of the three bouts. Blood samples were also obtained but at different intervals. Blood samples taken immediately before, immediately after, and thirty minutes after each bout. Data was analyzed with two-way ANOVA and bivariate correlations. Results showed three sequential bouts of heavy-resistance exercise increase serum TST and are effective at up-regulating AR mRNA and protein expression, which appears to correspond to subsequent increases in myofibril protein. Since an increase in TST, SHBG, FAI, skeletal muscle AR mRNA and protein expression, and myofibril protein content are known to increase muscle mass, these findings highlight the significance of sequential bouts of heavy-resistance exercise training for athletes looking to increase muscle mass.

Multiple Bouts of Heavy-Resistance Training Increases Muscle Mass

More research examining the effects of resistance training on the endocrine system looks to compare single-set versus multiple-set heavy-resistance exercise protocols influence on anabolic hormones. "Hormonal Responses of Multiset versus Single-Set Heavy-Resistance Exercise Protocols" (1997) took eight recreationally weight-trained men and had them complete two identical resistance exercise workouts one-set (1S) versus multiset (three sets [3S]). Researchers obtained blood work pre-exercise (PRE), immediately post-exercise (OP), and five minutes (5P), fifteen minutes (15P), thirty minutes (30P), and sixty minutes (60P) post-exercise and analyzed the samples for growth hormone (GH), testosterone (T), cortisol (C), and whole-blood lactate (L) levels. Results showed GH, L, and T significantly increased from PRE to OP in 1S and 3S and remained significantly elevated to 60P for 3S. Additionally, 3S showed significantly greater increases in GH, T, and L compared to 1S. For C increases were significant from resting at OP, 5P, and 15P for 3S and 1S; 3S increased compared to 1S at 5P, 15P, and 30P. The results show higher volumes of total-work produce significantly greater increases in circulating anabolic hormones during the recovery phase following exercise. For athletes who are constantly focusing on heavy-resistance training (heavy weight/low volume), it shows a place for high volume training (moderate weight/high volume) when attempting to increase anabolic hormones known to increase skeletal-muscle mass.

Heavy-Resistance and High-Volume Training Increase Anabolic Hormones

What about rest?

Rest period between sets is another significant training variable. Ahtiainen, Pakarinen, Alen, Kraemer, and Häkkinen (2005) set out to discover the influence short versus long rest periods between sets during resistance training have on muscle strength, size, and hormonal adaptions in trained men. Thirteen recreationally strength-trained men underwent a six-month hypertrophic strength-training period including two separate three-month training periods with the crossover design, a training protocol of short rest (SR, two minutes) versus long rest (LR, five minutes) between sets. At zero, three, and six months, basal hormonal concentrations of serum total testosterone (T), free testosterone (FT), and cortisol (C); dietary analysis; and muscle cross-sectional area (CSA) of the quadriceps femoris by magnetic resonance imagining (MRI) were measured. Maximal isometric strength of the leg extensors (right leg, one-repetition maximum) were also measured at zero, three, and six months under laboratory conditions.

Total volume of work (loads × sets × reps) were similar for both hypertrophic training protocols; however, intensity and the length of rest between sets varied; higher intensity and longer rest of five minutes versus somewhat lower intensity but shorter rest of two minutes. After the six-month training protocol was completed, data was gathered and analyzed using electromyographic (EMG) for maximal isometric force and blood samples for serum T, FT, C, and GH. Results showed no statistically significant difference between the two training protocols. This finding suggests both short-rest and long-rest intervals are acceptable for increasing muscle strength and size based on hormonal response. People adapt to the same stimulus in a variety of ways, this is why it is important to see what which combinations work best for you.

Heavy-Long-Rest & Moderate-Short-Rest Produce Anabolic Responses

Endurance training and hormonal responses

Moving away from endocrine response during resistance training and examining endurance training's effects on growth hormone, Weltman et al. (1992) set out to study intensity's effect on run training on the pulsatile release of growth hormone (GH) in twenty-one eumenorrheic untrained women. Participants were broken into three groups at-lactate threshold (/LT, n = 9), above-lactate threshold (greater than LT, n = 7), and the control group (n = 5). Measurements were taken for O_2 consumption (VO_2) at the lactate threshold (LT), fixed blood-lactate concentrations (FBLC) of 2.0, 2.5, and 4.0 mM, peak VO_2, maximal VO_2, body composition, and pulsatile release of GH. After a one-year period, results showed no change in the control group, subjects in both the /LT and greater than LT groups increased VO_2 and LT and FBLC of 2.0, 2.5, and 4.0 mM and VO_2max after one year of run training.

However, the increase observed in the greater than LT group was more than the /LT group. Body weight did not vary among- or within-group; however, percent body fat and fat weight did decrease in the greater than LT group and both training groups significantly increased fat-free weight. These findings suggest that endurance training both at-lactate threshold and above lactate threshold are effective methods of increasing lean tissue mass and reducing body fat. Above-lactate-threshold training displays greater lean tissue mass production and reduction of fat than at threshold training.

Training Above Lactate Threshold Increases Lean Mass & Fat Reduction

On males and aging

The following study by Roberts, Dalbo, Hassel, and Kerksick (2009) bridges the gap between younger and older men by examining aging and resistance exercise-related changes in intramuscular gene expression surrounding a single bout of resistance exercise. Participants completed 3 × 10 repetitions at 80 percent of their one-repetition maximum for Smith squat, leg press, and leg extension. Muscle biopsies were performed before and twenty-four hours after exercise, and venous blood was collected before, immediately after, and twenty-four hours after exercise. Findings revealed that free testosterone levels were greater in young participants at all-time points and even more so immediately following exercise. Pre-exercise growth hormone levels were similar for both groups, and both groups underwent an increase in growth hormone immediately post-exercise, with a greater increase occurring in the younger group. Older men displayed greater androgen-receptor levels at rest. A significant correlation was also noted between free-testosterone levels and basal androgen-receptor gene expression. Roberts and colleagues suggest these findings support androgen receptor expression patterns may be related to circulating free-testosterone levels. These finding may be the first step in unlocking gene-therapy techniques to increase free-testosterone levels and remedy muscle loss.

Free-Testosterone Levels Are Significant to Muscle Mass

"Testosterone and Growth Hormone Improve Body Composition and Muscle Performance in Older Men" (2009) tested the hypothesis that physiological supplementation with testosterone and GH together improve body composition and muscle performance of older men. Participants were one hundred twenty-two community-dwelling men 70.8 +/– 4.2 years of age. Participants were randomized to receive transdermal testosterone during a Leydig cell clamp plus GH for sixteen weeks. Data was collected using body composition by dual-energy x-ray absorptiometry, muscle performance, and safety test. Results showed lean body mass increase as did appendicular lean tissue. Total fat mass and trunk fat both decreased. Composite maximum-voluntary strength of upper and lower body muscles increased in the three highest dose groups, which correlated with changes in appendicular lean mass. Aerobic endurance increased in all six groups. Systolic and diastolic blood pressure increased similarly in each group. Those findings suggest that supplemental testosterone is an effective method for producing significant gains in total and appendicular lean mass, muscle strength, and aerobic endurance with significant reductions in whole-body trunk fat. Additionally, GH supplementation further enhanced those outcomes.

Specific to females

Progressing to studies concerning women, "The Effect of the Menstrual Cycle on Exercise Metabolism: Implications for Exercise Performance in Eumenorrhoeic Women" (2010) compiles research regarding female hormones estrogen and progesterone's relationship with exercise and athletic performance. Oosthuyse and Bosch (2010) found several studies revealing exercise performance and particularly endurance performance to vary between menstrual phases. With that said, the researchers also uncovered research claiming no such difference. Oosthuyse and Bosch conclude that the changes in performance during menstrual phase variations may be stimulated by the fluctuations in ovarian hormone concentrations.

The findings suggest estrogen may enhance endurance performance by altering carbohydrate, fat, and protein metabolism with progesterone acting antagonistically. Furthermore, estrogen improves short-term-duration exercise by promoting glucose availability and uptake into type I muscle fibers while progesterone inhibits these actions. Additionally, estrogen increases oxygen capacity in exercise as well as free fatty-acid availability. These findings and additional similar discoveries are justification for further investigation into female hormones estrogen and progesterone interactions with exercise during varying phases of the menstrual cycle.

Estrogen Enhances Endurance Performance

Dwelling deeper into the relationship between the different phases of the menstrual cycle and athletic performance is a study by Lebrun (1993) that looked at the effect of oral contraceptives on hormonal responses in relation to exercise. A survey on the menstrual cycle and performance indicated 37–63 percent of athletes did not report any cycle phase detriment, while 13–29 percent reported an improvement during menstruation. Lebrun notes there were small numbers of women studied making it difficult to interpret the numbers. It was also revealed that the best performances were typically during the immediate postmenstrual days and the wort performances during premenstrual phase and the first few days of menstrual flow. Swimmers were shown to improve performance during the menstrual phase and on the eighth day of the cycles and premenstrual worsening. Cross-country skiers recorded their best times during the postovulatory and postmenstrual phases. These findings suggest recommending training protocols according to cycle phase to achieve optimal performance. However, these results do display a bias because menstrual phase length and symptoms vary between women.

Overall

In brief, physical adaptions of the body resulting from exercise are not as straightforward as once thought. Endocrinology reveals there is more happening in the background than what superficial layers of exercise training present. Hormonal adaptions to exercise-training protocols, hormonal supplementation, age, and gender are all influenced by their interaction with the endocrine system. Further examination into the body's endocrine response to exercise related stimuli will revolutionize the exercise and sport industries. Science has only begun unlocking the physiology of exercise; as technology increases the human body can be studied under greater detail, and revolutionary discoveries can be made to change the way people participate in physical activity.

Every day it's the same routine, same intensity, for the same length of time, and yet you do not expect to walk away the same…insanity. "Insanity: doing the same thing repeatedly and expecting different results," said Albert Einstein.

What Are You Doing Differently Today to Get You Beyond Yesterday?

For your body to undergo change, it must adapt to a stress stimulus. This level of stress positively correlates to the amount of adaptation that will take place in your body postworkout. The greater the intensity of the workout, the stronger the adaptation response will be. The key is to cycle through hard days and easier recovery days rather than use the same level of intensity day after day. This will stimulate a greater training response while also allowing you to recover fully. It's a balancing act.

Everyone is different, so developing an individual athlete profile (assessments, training history, comparing competition results to norms, etc.) is the ideal way to figure out what works best for you. The important thing to remember is you need a workout hard enough to elicit a strong adaptation response but not so hard that you cannot recover within the day or two you have before your next hard effort. If you train too hard, then you will not fully recover and not be able to workout at maximum capacity.

Moreover, you will start your adaptation response from a lower point, consequently not improving as much as possible. You want to be fully recovered between hard efforts but not take so much time between them that you lose out on the frequency and volume of hard sessions. It's a delicate balance. These same fluctuations in intensity need to be seen on the big scale as well (weeks, months, years).

How Much Is Enough?

PROformance Training Systems Exercise Recommendation Chart					
Type of Activity		Lose Ability	Maintain Ability	Gain Ability	Activity Duration
Mechanical	Metabolic	Training Frequency (Days Per Week)			Minutes
Basic Mobility and Strength	Weight Control/ Maintenance	1–2	3	4–5	30
Hypertrophy (Muscle Size)	Competitive Endurance	<3	3–4	5–6	45–90
Athletic Strength	Competitive Conditioning (Non-Endurance Athletes)	1–2	3	4–5	45–60
Competitive Power	Basic Cardiovascular Health	1	2	3–4	30–45

The purpose of this chart is to show you what it takes to lose, maintain, and gain ability in specific areas of fitness. Mechanical and metabolic activities are listed next to each other making it easier to read the chart; they are not listed in this manner to imply which training focuses should be paired.

Types of activity can overlap for a given day. For instance, basic mobility and strength can be performed between sets focusing on competitive power on the same day. This allows for the best use of time while improving upon all types of activity. Don't become confused by the two segregated columns "mechanical" and "metabolic" on the PTS Progression Model. Mechanical and metabolic training can and often will occur concurrently such as during high-intensity interval training (HIIT). The combination of the two systems just needs to be appropriately matched up with the athlete's stage of development. On the next page is a one-day training journal that can be copied and used for logging progress, feel free to make as many copies of the next page (and only the next page) as you like.

It's A Combination of Hard Hard-Days and Easy Easy-Days That Lead to Adaption

Mechanical Theme

Mob. > Corr. > Func. Stability > NM Efficiency > Muscular Endurance > Hypertrophy > Heavy Power > Max Power > AMS.

Metabolic Theme

Met. Stim. > Aero. Elevation > Thresh. Development > Aero. Capacity > An. Expansion > Spec. Movements > Spec. Skills

Date	Warm-Up		Cooldown		Primary Focus Movements
	Exercise	*Duration*	*Exercise*	*Duration*	Knee Hinge
__/__/__					Hip Hinge
					Vertical Push
					Vertical Pull
					Horizontal Push
					Horizontal Pull
					Core

Activity	Sets	Reps/Time	Weight/Distance	Rest

If you want to improve, you must train using a progression system. As the last chapter mentioned, it is during the resting period after you exercise that your body improves. Now let's take this a little further. The workload your body went through during exercise was a stimulus that your body reacted to by adapting (improving) to during your rest period. Your body was given something it could not fully handle, so it adapted making next session slightly easier.

Remember how I mentioned earlier, humans are creatures of extreme efficiency? As a result, we adapt our body making ourselves more efficient, but what happens when your body is fully adapted to the workout it is given? Nothing. Nothing as in, it ceases to further adapt to the stimulus because your body has already adapted to the stimulus. This means you will no longer continue to jump higher, run further, or lift more because you have not challenged your body.

What this means to you as the athlete is there needs to be a new stimulus added to your routine. This stimulus can be any variety of things from a different weight and reps scheme, to shorter rest, or to completely new exercises. That is decided based upon what you have been doing and your goals. With that said, one thing is always constant; to keep seeing improvements, nothing can be constant. Different variables always need to be changing throughout your workouts for your body to have a new adaption stimulus.

Adaption is The Accord Between Repeated Exposure and Frequent Change

In view of that, you must always keep an eye on your workouts making sure to alter something every session. Don't change every aspect, because your body does need time to adapt. But rather keep your workout planned one step ahead so that as soon as you adapt to one stimulus, there is another challenge awaiting.

We live in a society of maximizing efficiency. When it comes to our fitness routines, there is no difference. Every day we log on to our favorite news site, see the latest time-efficient workout craze, read it, and say one of two things:

1. "This workout is impossible!"
2. "I don't have time for this workout!"

Don't worry, I don't have time for fads either, so rather than writing a book about the next three-month long fitness craze, I would like to share with you how to filter through the junk. Let's go over a little bit behind the basics of energy expenditure, so we can learn how to further challenge ourselves by altering the terrain we perform our favorite activities on, spending more time doing what we enjoy while improving our workouts.

First, energy expenditure is simply the amount of energy being expended during a given activity. The more systemic (whole body) the activity is, the more muscles are being used, meaning more oxygen needs to be delivered to those muscles, meaning the heart needs to pump faster, and thus we need more energy (calories) to get and keep this entire process moving.

Systemic > Increased Active Musculature > More Required Blood Flow > Increased Heart Rate > Higher Energy Expenditure

The best way to think of this is exercises using more overall bodily movement require more calories in general. This is evident in running's or hiking's greater energy expenditure than cycling or walking. Now, this is all true for the same effort. If a runner is going for a light jog on a level street and a cyclist is killing it on an uphill, then the cyclist will crush the runner in terms of energy expenditure due to the increased demand of her environment (the slope increase of the hill).

Using the terrain as a variable in energy expenditure is a tool you can use to increase exercise demand. Stable environments require less energy expenditure. For instance, walking on pavement requires less energy than walking on packed snow in the woods. This is because walking on packed snow requires more synergist muscles (supporting muscles) to support you on the uneven terrain. Take this a step further, walking on sand demands even more support and energy expenditure than walking on packed snow.

If we want to increase our energy expenditure and further challenge our body, mind, and spirit, then change your terrain. Changing your terrain adds benefits beyond energy expenditure. Run across the beach rather than on pavement. Switch up road cycling with mountain biking. Try open water swimming instead of the pool (only if you are a strong and experienced swimmer with a partner). Ski cross-country as opposed to downhill. These changes not only alter energy expenditure, strength, and proprioception development, but they also change your scenery, atmosphere, social scene, and mind-set.

You're coming up to the home stretch of your race, and you're running on empty. You feel as if the finish will never come, or if it does, it will be with you in a stretcher. Then suddenly you get this surge of energy blasting you through the finish. Sound familiar? If it does, then you're like many people who get psyched up by the distance they just covered in their race and start to bonk only to sprint to the finish when it's in sight. Why does this phenomenon occur and what can we do to overcome it?

A popular belief as to why this "psych-out bonk" occurs is because our body's natural set points for the distance we are attempting based upon experience with the distance are telling our brain that we are going way too hard for this distance, so slow down the pace (Tucker and Dugas 2009). This holds true even when you have practiced the distance numerous times, because every time we race, we are pushing our bodies beyond what practice requires. However, the more you race the distance, the more adapt to these faster race checkpoints your body becomes, thus lowering your body's level of "psych-out bonk." Besides the obvious training at race pace to overcome this empty tank sensation at the end of your race, the best method I have come up with to keep your body going smooth and strong to the finish is with positive affirmation.

Positive affirmation is a form of mental sports coaching. It incorporates telling and convincing yourself that you have successfully accomplished this race distance before at this pace, and you are about to do it again. It is both helpful and important to tell yourself this during your race, even if you have not yet accomplished the feat because you will fool your mind into believing you have done it successfully in the past even if you have not, getting you to the finish strong.

Positive Affirmation is Mind Over Matter

Positive affirmation is useful during all sports. First championship game? "I'm already a champion." Recovering from injury? "I've come back from worse." Keep missing your shot? "I've made this shot one thousand times before." Regardless of the sport or mental block, positive affirmation can help.

Positive Affirmation Will Help You in all Areas of Life

Practice telling yourself these positive affirmations daily before, during, and after practice. Learn that believing in yourself (and reminding yourself through positive affirmation about these beliefs) is the key to success in any endeavor whether athletic or not.

Additionally, use imagery techniques to immerse yourself in the situation. Imagery is a sport psychology tool used for visualizing yourself performing your sport exactly how you want it to play out during competition. It can also be used for visualizing how you will deal with setbacks and obstacles. For imagery to work best, visualize yourself in competition through the first-person perspective. Visualize your opponents, how you interact with your team, how every movement feels, distinctive smells, the texture of your equipment, and anything else that can make the scenario more real. The mind cannot tell the difference between an activity you performed and one you visualized. Knowing this, use imagery paired with positive affirmation to break mental barriers, set new personal records, and beat the competition.

The Mind Cannot Tell the Difference Between Visualization Techniques and Reality

During my time in the sports and fitness industry, I have seen a lot of different techniques—some of which are good and some not so good. Most of them have a certain purpose with hopes of producing a desired outcome. Others are used just because they are "sexy exercises." What I mean by sexy exercises is exercises that hold no true value to the outcome of the athlete's goals but rather look cool and interesting for the sake of selling a new fitness product or training service. Maybe it is an exercise or routine that an athlete reads about in a magazine and is now fixated on. It is for this reason that background checks on your coach should be performed to ensure adequate education and experience. Both education and experience are important for good coaching, because as the saying goes, theory and practice are always the same in theory but never in practice. By choosing a coach with exposure to both, it will lessen this divide.

When working with an athlete, he puts his performance in the coach or trainer's hands. It is in turn the coach's duty to ensure the highest probability of a successful outcome during the athlete's primary exhibition. Although athletes should look forward to their training, it is not the coach's responsibility to make the workout look impressive to entertain the athlete with trending exercises simply because they are in style. Nonetheless, far too often this is the case with new and inexperienced coaches and trainers. Coaches, please remind your athletes that individual training sessions are not meant to impress them, but are rather the result of reaching their season and career long goals. Knowing that, if you are a coach and you feel your athletes will quit if you don't give them the trendy exercises they want because other coaches are employing them, then use other methods to make your sessions fun! Keeping clients engaged is part of the art of coaching. Study gamification and apply its techniques to your sessions. This is why during PTS we always monitor and adjust workouts, so we have appropriate exercise selection. Athletes, remember you are training to aspire towards excellence. It's not always going to be enjoyable, matter of fact, it will often be temporary discomfort in exchange for long-term victory.

With that said, "keep it simple stupid" (KISS). Far too often these fancy exercises are too overwhelming for the athlete attempting them. This leads to compensations, and when the body reaches a compensatory state, it results in altered neuromuscular control (controlling the body as it moves), which in turn leads to musculoskeletal disorders (injuries to muscles and/or bones). What this means is back off on your sexy exercises and keep them simple. Take time to adapt to the "boring" exercises, so when it is time to systematically progress to the next progression, you can do so without compensation and thus achieve the desired outcome.

The best military plan is usually the simplest one. The same goes for sports and fitness. Do what has known to work for decades, not what some celebrity trainer made up last night. There is reason why certain exercise techniques from the seventies and eighties and even earlier are coming back into style, because although people got bored of them, they worked. There are also reasons why certain exercises never faded out of style—they work. Do yourself a favor the next time you're at the gym and debating between a new trendy workout and a simple time-tested workout, keep it simple.

Make a Simple Plan and Execute

How many times have you heard the expression "practice makes perfect?" Unfortunately, I am not going to tell you that was all a lie and give you a way around it. Instead I am going to explain why it works and why you should continue practicing.

It takes over ten thousand repetitions of a movement to "master" it. Now that is a lot of steps, hang cleans, snatches, and so on. During this process, your body is learning new patterns between motor neurons (specialized cells that pass signals to target cells) and synapses (the gateway that motor neurons pass through) allowing it to perform actions quicker, smoother, and more efficiently. Over time, your body will eventually develop what is known as reflexive intelligence.

Reflexive intelligence is when you don't even realize you are doing it right—it's just natural. And that is what separates the average Joe from the D1 superstar or professional athlete. Reflexive intelligence, the ability to just make it happen. Practice is repetition, and repetition leads to habit, which makes things come naturally. Knowing this, the repetitions must be deliberate, well-planned actions. Practicing a movement ten thousand times improperly will not do you any good. Find a qualified coach and learn how to properly execute the movements.

Reflexive Intelligence is What Allows Us to Perform Without Thinking

In the Army, we endlessly practice warrior task and battle drills, so they become second nature. Warrior task and battle drills are how we operate as a team and as individuals within a team during operations. By repeatedly practicing what we need to do, when the time comes and it is a stressful situation, reflexive intelligence kicks in and we instinctively act out the patterns we learn.

Like I said, I have no secret for you to make this easier. Just keep practicing and remember, the reason why the pros make it look so easy is because they put in all the work rather than complaining about having to go to practice; they don't whine and quit when they get out kicked at the finish. They understand that if they want to be a track or football star, then there is a job to be done. There are no true "free rides" in sports.

Mechanical Training

Stages of Mechanical Training

I break down mechanical training into six stages, corrective, stabilization, muscular endurance, hypertrophy/strength, heavy power, and max power. Although these stages can be trained concurrently during a single training session, each session must focus on which stage and larger theme you want to improve. If you are not focused on your goal, your program will be all over the map and limited progress will be made.

Corrective Exercise: Work on any muscle imbalances and/or joint dysfunctions that may have occurred during the previous season.

» *Myofascial Release:* Thirty-second holds on tight/overactive muscles including proprioceptive neuromuscular facilitation (PNF) and self-myofascial release (SMR).

» *Resistance Training:* Two to three sets of twelve to fifteen repetitions with sixty-second rest at 40–60 percent 1RM.

Stabilization Training: Introduce exercises on unstable yet controlled surfaces such as wobble boards, balance pads, split stance, and single leg stance. This will enhance your body's proprioception, balance, and firing order and rate. Your body will learn to use its stabilizing muscles better to assist the prime movers, which will lead to greater strength and power development during the later stages of training.

» *Resistance Training:* Three sets of twelve to fifteen repetitions with thirty- to forty-five-second rest at 50–70 percent 1RM.

Muscular Endurance Training: Implement high-repetitions, short-rest resistance training with relatively light weight to enhance muscular endurance and increase sarcoplasmic hypertrophy.

» *Resistance Training:* Three sets of twelve to fifteen repetitions with thirty-second rest at 50–75 percent 1RM.

Hypertrophy/Strength Training: Drop down the repetitions and up the resistance to enhance strength gains while still developing upon muscular endurance by initiating cross-sectional growth and further developing the sarcoplasm (part of the cell containing "fuel" for contraction).

» *Resistance Training:* Three to four sets of six to twelve repetitions with 45–120-second rest at 75–85 percent 1RM.

Heavy Power Training: Develop the ability to generate high levels of force by lifting extremely demanding loads with complete rest for maximum motor recruitment and force development.

» *Resistance Training:* Five to six sets of one to five repetitions with three- to five-minute rest at 85–100 percent 1RM.

Max Power Training: Insert the speed component to the Power = Force × Speed equation to add the finishing touch to your resistance training. This is moving lighter loads as fast and safely as possible.

» *Resistance Training:* Three to six sets of one to ten repetitions with three- to five-minute rest at 30–45 percent 1RM or 10 percent body weight.

Stages of Mechanical Training Composition

Mechanical Training Progression				
Method of Training	**Sets**	**Reps**	**Rest (s)**	**%1RM**
Corrective	2–3	12–15	60	40–60
Stabilization	3	12–15	30–45	50–70
Muscular Endurance	3	12–15	Up to 30	50–75
Hypertrophy/Strength	3–4	6–12	45–120	75–85
Heavy Power	5–6	1–5	180–300	85–100
Max Power	3–6	1–10	180–300	30–45 or 10% BW

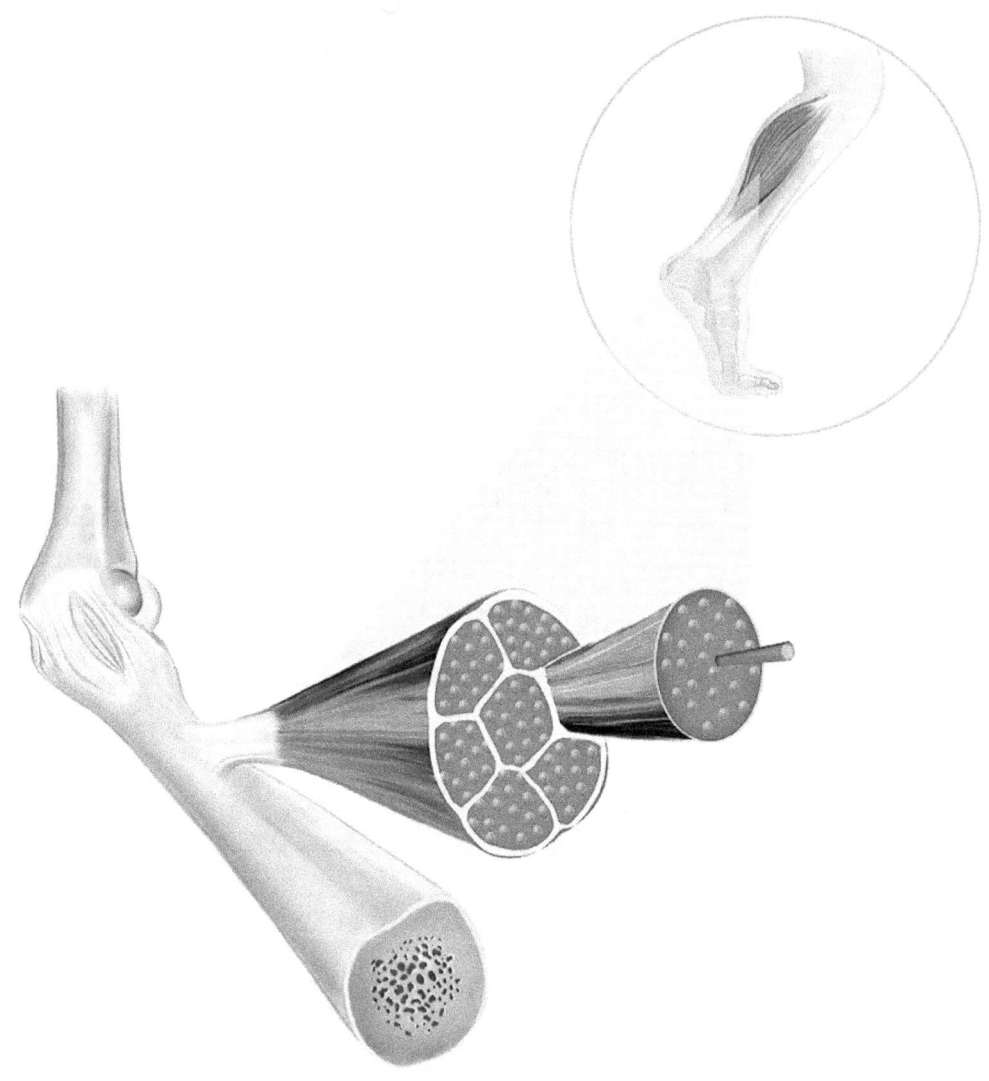

To get bigger, faster, and stronger, you need to build more muscle through resistance training. Do you know what is going on in your muscles that make you bigger, faster, and stronger? Here is a cross-sectional illustration of the inside of your calf muscle (gastrocnemius), from the fiber down to the sarcomere. A sarcomere is the most basic part of a muscle, containing the contractile filaments.

Muscles adapt in two ways. First, the cross-sectional fibers (myofibrils or contractile proteins) of your muscles get micro tears from the stress of moving heavy loads, adapting and thickening the myofibrils by activating satellite cells and transforming them into new contractile filaments. This results in more connection points for them to pull upon the next time you attempt to move a resistance. Your muscles are "calling for backup." This occurs during repetitions above 85% of your 1RM (repetition max).

The second way your muscles adapt involves the sarcoplasmic reticulum. This fluid filled area surrounding the muscle becomes "flooded" with metabolic sources from high-volume, short-rest exercise using moderate resistance. Specific metabolic sources are ATP/CP, glucose, creatine, calcium, and water, and they are there to supply the cross-sectional fibers with energy and contraction/reaction enzymes. This is what causes the pump/swelling effect in muscles when you are performing hypertrophy and endurance-training workouts. When the sarcoplasmic reticulum becomes engorged with these metabolic sources of energy and enzymes, it is storing more fuel for your next workout. The muscle "realizes" it became depleted because it did not store enough fuel the last time, so it adapted and will store more for the next time, resulting in muscle growth (hypertrophy). This occurs with rest periods lasting less than thirty seconds.

Those are the two means by which muscles are built. One mechanism enhances contractile ability and the other increases efficiency. By working both systems, heavy and low repetition with long rest and moderate and high repetition with short rest, we can enhance the athletic ability of both, making us faster and stronger athletes.

Skeletal Muscle Structure

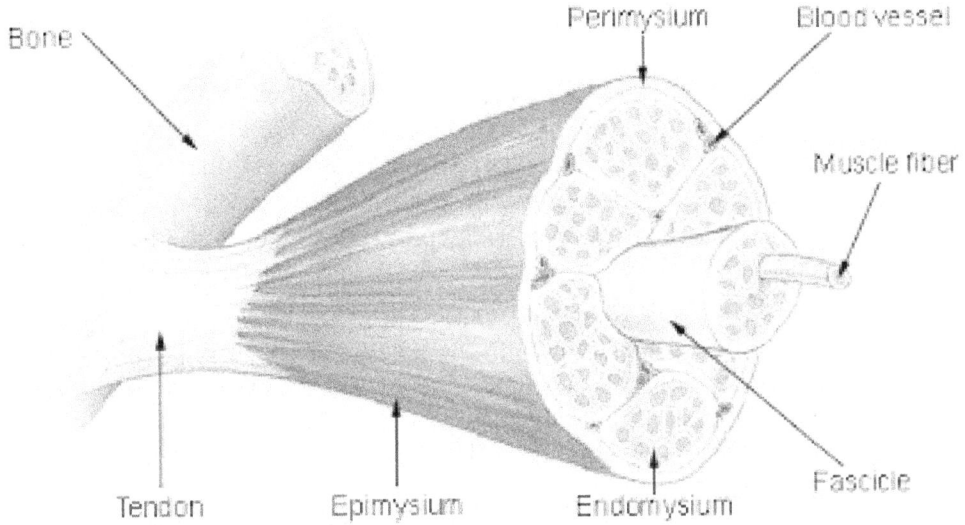

Fascia keeps the body stabilized. If you know anything about fascia, it is probably that fascia covers and connects everything in the body. But did you know that it does this in just one sheath? That's right; your plantar fascia, fascia covering your biceps, and even fascia covering your brain are all part of the same sheath with no interruptions.

For that reason, the body can never work in isolation. Whenever you pull or shorten fascia in one area, you affect it in another area; this is known as spiraling fascia. Cutting-edge coaches are training elite-level sprinters to twist their wrist in certain motions (supination and pronation) to influence the fascia at their hips. That's right; a flick of the wrist really can make a difference in a sprinter's career, at least for Tyson Gay when he beat Usain Bolt after training using spiraling for his fascia. Do I have your attention now?

Fascial Training Improves Power and Speed

So how does it all work? Fascia is still relatively new to the world of exercise and sport science, but the research we do have revealed fascia having ten times more sensory neurons than muscle, meaning there needs to be some focus on fascial training as well as neuromusculoskeletal training. This can be achieved by performing counter-movements (small quick movements in the opposite direction of the desired motion) prior to the primary action of the muscle. Reason being, fascia has highly elastic properties; therefore, it responds well to stretching.

Fascia has many neurons and elastic properties; it also acts as a hybrid for muscles. Studies show that the stretch of the fascia aids in energy output when released, as the muscles isometrically and concentrically contract. Meaning, less energy needs to be used by your body because it is being applied by the fascia as stored and released elastic energy. What this means to you is when you train your fascia more efficiently, it will help reduce your energy needs, saving energy for later in your workout.

Thomas Myers in his *Anatomy Trains* system declares twelve "myofascial meridians" unifying sections of muscle through fascia. These myofascial lines are the planes which movement mainly occurs and are:

1. The Superficial Front Line
2. The Superficial Back Line
3. The Lateral Line (Front & Back)
4. Back Functional Line
5. Front Functional Line
6. Spiral Line
7. Deep Front Line (Lower Anterior & Upper Posterior)
8. Deep Front Line (Upper Middle & Upper Anterior)
9. Deep Front Arm Line
10. Superficial Front Arm Line
11. Deep Back Arm Line
12. Superficial Back Arm Line

Think of the lines as highways which movement moves more fluid and energy transfers throughout the body most efficiently. I would suggest reading Myer's book to grasp the full concept. I am only mentioning myofascial lines to illustrate how the body operates holistically in one great sheath rather than in isolation by individual muscles.

Building upon that, keep variety in your workouts. Life never follows the same repetitive pattern, so why should practice? Remember to vary your reps, weight, rest, duration, frequency, and intensity on a regular basis. Fascia needs to adapt to a variety of pulls in numerous directions with varying intensities to function most efficiently. The best way to do that is to simply add variety.

When you are making your exercise selection, what are the ways you go about doing so? Do you pick a body part you feel needs attention, and then choose an exercise working the desired region? If you said yes, then you are in the same boat as the clear majority of people who are still training in the dark ages. If you said no, then great! You can stop reading because I'm only going to tell you what you already know.

As I previously mentioned, the body in all its complexity is simple. What I mean is although the body is an amazing piece of overwhelming complexity, it does not even know what a muscle is. Yeah, that's right. Although the body could not move without muscles, it does not even know what muscles are. But that is OK, because the body does not need to understand what muscles are. It needs to know movement. The body is concerned with movement, not muscles, so stop basing your program design around certain muscles and start designing it around specific movements. The body almost never works in isolation; it works in integrated movements. With that said, train (or teach) it that way. Train (teach) the body to improve what it does, move.

There is a sea creature known as a Sea Squirt that metabolizes or "eats" its brain upon completing its larva (infant) stage since it has found its home and no longer needs its tadpole like anatomy to move. What this tells us is our brain's primary function is movement, there is a clear relationship between our body and mind and movement is that connection.

If you want to become better at anything involving movement and are looking toward exercise as a means of getting you there (this is usually a good idea), then stop thinking of the body in isolated parts, and start referring to it as one integrated system. Determine the primary movements of your goal and progressively mimic them in slightly altered variations. By using slight variations of an exercise in successive workouts, it adds a stress to the body that it will adapt to over time.

Properly Executing Movement Patterns is Essential for Athletic Success

Ten basic movements that should be kept in mind when designing a program are:
1. Walk/Run
2. Squat
3. Lunge
4. Hip Hinge
5. Vertical Push
6. Horizontal Push
7. Vertical Pull
8. Horizontal Pull
9. Rotation
10. Anti-Rotation

Athletic development is essential for success in any sport. Regardless of the objective of the sport or the fine motor skills involved, all sports involve some degree of developing gross motor skills. In the last few years there has been a growing interest in methods used to increase athletic development. Quite recently, considerable attention has been paid to neuromuscular training such as plyometrics, proprioception, pliability, and sprint ability as essential ingredients in athletic success. Having said that, athletes and coaches are continuously searching for new marvels in training that are going to drive them to heightened levels of excellence.

This chapter discusses specific fundamentals of athletic development, power, neuromuscular efficiency, and sprint ability. These attributes of athleticism play a vital role in the success of an athlete, as well as are key elements of sport-specific skill development. Beginning by giving a comprehensive account of traditional research aiming to improve upon athletic development and then going back to analyze these findings, here are the topics we will cover:

1. Focusing on methods of improving vertical jump performance, which is thought of as the leading predictor of power (Ostoji´c, Stojanovi´c, Ahmetovi´c 2010).
2. The benefits of plyometric training on numerous athletic variables.
3. Neuromuscular and proprioception trainings' effect on injury prevention.
4. A comparison between plyometric training and stabilization/balance training.
5. Sprint training as an advantageous and time-efficient training method.

Vertical jump

Jump performance, specifically vertical jump height, is widely used as the main predictor of raw power in sports. The vertical jump displays the ability for an individual to propel her body straight-up against gravity. Vertical jump testing is straightforward and highly correlates with relative power production (Ostoji´c, Stojanovi´c, Ahmetovi´c 2010). With that said, the focus of recent research has been on improving vertical jump height through maximal heavy-resistance, maximal-power, and plyometric training (Andrew et al. 2010; de Villarreal, Izquierdo, & Gonzalez-Badilo 2011; Markovic 2007; Tricoli et al. 2005; Wisløff et al. 2004). Findings of this research show vertical jump height is sensitive to other training modalities.

The results of the research on improving vertical jump height through maximal heavy-resistance, maximal-power, and plyometric training have shown both traditional slow-velocity strength training such as half squats as well as faster power-oriented strength training such as plyometrics and Olympic weightlifting are successful at improving vertical jump ability both alone and when combined (Andrew et al. 2010; de Villarreal, Izquierdo, and Gonzalez-Badilo 2011; Markovic 2007; Tricoli et al. 2005; Wisløff et al. 2004). These findings are due to a neuromuscular adaption resulting in a reduction in time for the firing rate at which the contractile filaments are able to contract as well as the amount of force produced under the given load that is the athlete's weight. The combination of these two elements leads to an increase in power output measurable by vertical jump height.

Vertical Jump Height is the Gold Standard of Measuring Power Output

Out of all the athlete training methods, perhaps the most highly transferable to athletic skills is plyometrics. Although strength and power training produce the work capacity necessary to perform athletic movements, plyometric training transfers that force and power to sport specific skills. For several years, great effort has been devoted to the study of the neuromuscular implications that plyometric training has on muscle fiber characteristics, power output, force production, and agility. In general, an accumulation of research on plyometrics has shown plyometric training to be exceptionally advantageous to athletes desiring to increase these athletic parameters (Markovic et al. 2007; Miller et al. 2006; Potteiger et al. 1999; Wilson, Murphy, and Giorgi 1996).

Findings on the research regarding plyometric training on enhancing athletic parameters indicate that plyometric training is effective at improving agility performance after only six weeks of training (Miller et al. 2006). Plyometric training also increased power output that may be a result of increased muscle size (Potteiger et al. 1999). As well as an improvement in eccentric contractibility beyond that of what weight-training provides (Wilson, Murphy, and Giorgi 1996). Since vertical jump height is a descendent of plyometric training, the training adaptions seen in plyometric training are similar but not limited to vertical jump height. Plyometric training can result in an increase in lateral movement, agility, and sprint ability due to the neuromuscular adaptions occurring during the specific exercise.

Six Weeks of Plyometric Training Show an Improvement in Athletic Ability

Neuromuscular and proprioception training for injury prevention

Several publications have appeared in recent years documenting the effectiveness of neuromuscular and proprioception training on injury prevention. Research has suggested neuromuscular and proprioception training as effective applications of an injury-prevention training program in athletes from a range of backgrounds participating in a range of sports and focusing on varying areas of the body (Holm et al. 2004; Pánics et al. 2008; Zebis et al. 2008).

Injury prevention plays an important role in athletic development. Specifically, neuromuscular training in the form of proprioception training has shown its effectiveness in preventing injuries in knees (Pánics et al. 2008; Zebis et al. 2008). Additionally, those same injury-prevention programs implemented to prevent knee injuries have also been shown to improve dynamic balance in athletes (Holm et al. 2004). For this reason, the implementation of proprioception training into an athlete's training regimen is beneficial for athletes desiring to increase performance as well as hoard off injuries. By providing athletes with full-bodied workouts aimed at improving all areas of athletic performance, it decreases their chances of injury while improving athletic success.

Knee Injury Prevention Programs Should be Included Throughout Programing

Plyometric vs. stabilization training

In the literature, several theories have proposed to explain what is better for improving athletic performance, high-intensity training or stabilization and balance training. Two significant articles look directly at this question, asking what are the effects of plyometric training versus dynamic stabilization training on a multitude of athletic variables? In the end, plyometric and stabilization/balance training were shown to be equally important at improving athletic development and should both be included in injury prevention and preseason programs among athletes, supplementing their strengths and weaknesses (Myer et al. 2006a, 2006b).

Programs must Include Plyometric and Stabilization Exercises for Optimal Results

The value of sprint performance

Sprint performance is extensively studied because of its influence in athletic performance. The ability to accelerate quickly and acquire a relatively high speed is dependent on many factors from skeletal muscle composition, oxidative capacity, metabolism, as well as other long-term metabolic adaptions. Previous research has demonstrated that sprint interval training is as effective or better at enhancing these parameters than other training modalities (Burgomaster, Heigenhauser, and Gibala1985; Burgomaster et al. 2008; Burgomaster et al. 2005; Duncan et al. 2005; Markovic et al. 2007; Ross and Leveritt 2001).

The findings on sprint performance indicate sprinting is just as effective if not more effective at improving athletic performance than plyometric training (Markovic et al. 2007). Furthermore, sprint intervals have been shown to be as effective as endurance training with the added benefit of time-efficiency (Burgomaster, Heigenhauser, and Gibala 2006; Burgomaster et al. 2008; Burgomaster et al. 2005; Duncan et al. 2005; Ross and Leveritt 2001). These findings suggest sprint training as an effective and efficient strategy for increasing athletic development. One of the greatest challenges of training athletes today is incorporating the most effective training program that is also time-efficient. Sprinting as the findings show appears to be a very appropriate method for achieving this goal.

Sprint Training is an Effective and Efficient Substitute for Plyometric Training

Overall

Athletic development cannot be attributed to any one mechanism. Training an athlete involves progressing the athlete across a spectrum of athletic focuses (themes in PTS) aimed at different functions but with the same primary goal to make the athlete more functional in her given sport. Power is a vital element of many sports. With that said, vertical jump height is widely considered the golden standard of lower-body power-production measurement. Knowing this, tremendous effort should be placed on exercises improving vertical jump height. Since vertical jump height is a product of power-to-weight ratio, attention should be placed on strategies enhancing explosive power without adding unwanted bulk. Plyometric training is an excellent method of accomplishing this because of plyometrics focus on quick movements that are typically performed at body weight or with relatively light loads still allowing the athlete to move quickly without producing levels of muscle hypertrophy that can reduce her power-to-weight ratio and hinder her explosiveness and ability to perform the skills of her sport quickly.

Plyometric training shows promise in pure applicable power. Plyometrics take speed training and apply it under a variety of different axis, forces, and rates to best simulate those elements found in sport. Furthermore, heavy-strength and explosive-power training have been shown to effectively improve plyometric ability by altering muscle fiber characteristics, increasing muscle size, and improving firing rate. These metabolic adaptions allow athletes to get more from their sport. Keeping in mind plyometrics is an umbrella covering several neuromuscular actions that occur at a high rate, plyometrics include variations of the vertical jump such as depth-jump, one-legged vertical jump, two-legged vertical jump, as well as horizontal bounding. These jumping drills as well as numerous agility drills utilizing cutting and agility maneuvers aid in the athletic development of athletes by improving the transfer between exercise and athletic skill.

Plyometrics Increase Pure Applicable Power

With the above sections focusing primarily on high-intensity aspects of neuromuscular training, effort should be taken to highlight the vital role balance and stability play in controlling athletes' movements. Findings show that proprioception exercises focusing on balance and stability provide benefits that supplement plyometric training, allowing the athlete to perform at a higher level, while also reducing injury risk. Balance and stability exercises add control to athletic development that other training methods do not achieve as well. This added level of control improves performance in high-intensity exercise, improving overall athletic performance.

Current research on athletic development has shown tremendous benefits of power, strength, plyometric, and balance/stability training. However, which single training method produces the best results is still unanswered. Although all areas of training focus on different aspect of performance funneling together to create a better performing athlete, sprint training has been shown to be as effective of a method as the other modes of training at increasing athletic development in a variety of areas, since sprint training involves producing power at a high rate while efficiently propelling the body forward by utilizing high levels of proprioception, sprinting has been shown to be an effective blend of exercise-training methods. With that said, sprint training should not be overlooked as a noteworthy exercise for improving athletic performance regardless of how simple and novice the exercise may appear.

Sprinting is a Harmony of Explosive Power and Delicate Proprioception

From the outcome of our investigation, it is possible to conclude that athletic development is a complex and complicated phenomenon. Due to the varying degree of elements involved in athletic development, ranging from the demands of a sport to the abilities and needs of an individual athlete, it is essential that athletes and coaches have a sound understanding of all the exercises involved in engineering a mechanically sound athlete, how to improve and progress upon those exercises, and what those exercises and training focuses do for the athletes that are relevant to their goals. To ensure the best possible product, athletes and coaches must establish a training regimen that best encompasses all the elements of an optimally performing athlete. What constitutes an optimally performing athlete depends on the athlete's needs, abilities, and desires. Careful attention should be placed on what training method is best to produce a desired result as well as what supplemental training method best compliments the primary method to compound athletic progress. Overall, it is easy to see how an activity that appears as simple as choosing an exercise is exceedingly intricate and needs to be constructed under a careful eye with a knowledgeable mind and thoughtful attention.

With that said, this is the exact reason PTS was developed. Any strength coach or personal trainer claiming to have the best training is ill-informed. PROformance Training Systems is a system explaining one technique of developing an athlete but leaves the method up to the athlete and coach. There are hundreds of training styles out there, I am simply attempting to give you guidance in how to pair those styles and in which order I recommend they be performed.

Runners tend to rely heavily on their cardiovascular system to do all the work, rarely thinking about the muscular system's role in distance-running success. Regardless of what we may think, our muscular system plays just as vital of a role to our running pace as our heart and lungs.

Think about this, the stronger our running muscles are, the more force they can produce at a given speed, and thus the faster we can run while using less energy. Put another way,

More Strength → More Force Production = More Speed with Reduced Energy Use
=
Faster Overall Pace with Less Effort

Strength development is primarily a result of overcoming a resistance, not increasing speed. The more force we must generate to overcome a resistance, the stronger we become. Knowing this, let's focus on increasing strength through running for a moment. Running faster increases the amount of fibers activated but only to a degree. We recruit additional muscle fibers in a process known as The Motor Unit Recruitment Ladder. Basically, we begin on the lowest rung of the ladder, type I (slow twitch fibers) and recruit faster activating muscle fibers that can handle a higher intensity as we go up the ladder (type IIa and type IIb). Intensity can be force, speed, or fatigue, and the rate we move up the ladder depends on that intensity. Although an individual's personal VO_2max required to activate a given muscle fiber (slow or fast twitch) varies with running ability, the percent VO_2max that a fiber is activated is relatively constant from person to person.

Motor Unit Recruitment Ladder

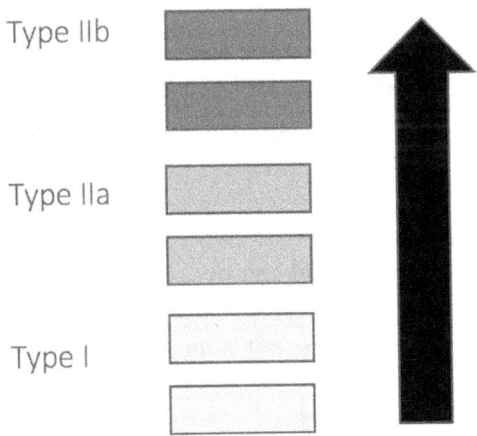

Type IIb

Type IIa

Type I

This means the type of running workouts we choose not only affects our cardiovascular system but also our muscular system. Therefore, muscle activation and recruitment must be brought into consideration when designing a training program.

In addition to the number of fibers activated, once the specific fiber type reaches its upper limit or ability to produce force, it begins to fire at a faster rate (more twitches per minute). This is done because the body naturally wants to work as efficiently as possible, by using fewer fibers at a faster rate as opposed to activating more fibers. Think of the process as being a supervisor and having employees at work. It is cheaper to have fewer employees working harder than to bring more employees on shift. That is however, until a certain point. At that point, we must bring in more employees before the employees cease to work and the whole job stops.

Muscle Fiber-Type Activation Thresholds

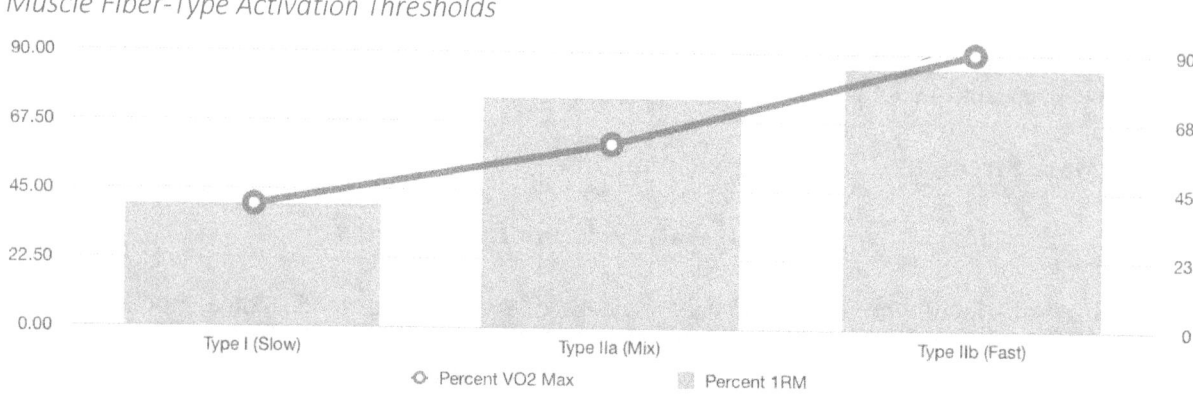

It is for this reason we have to work on plyometric exercises that improve muscle firing rate, as well as speed work on the track to improve the speed of our contractions and improve leg turnover. These quick movement exercises teach our opposing muscles how to switch roles as the agonist muscle switches roles (the front and back of your thigh's muscles cannot both shorten and at the same time). Or to stick with our employee analogy, only one employee can work at a station at a time or they will get in each other's way and slow down the process. This is known as reciprocal inhibition and is improved by challenging it with speed for advanced runners and basic proprioception exercises for novices.

Plyometrics Improve Reciprocal Inhibition

That said, pure resistance training via free weights and short-hill sprints (up to ten seconds) is the best way to train for max force development and should be a key part in the runner's training program if they wish to take full advantage of improved running through increased max strength. Nevertheless, runners should implement short intervals on a track and explosive running drills to amplify the crossover to distance running.

As I mentioned, plyometrics are another asset to a runner's success. They not only provide force for strength development but increase effectiveness by enhancing neuromuscular efficiency (communication between the muscles and nervous system). This allows the drills to act as both the force component and speed component, giving them a great appeal to distance runners.

Knee Lift and Heel Tuck to Improve Running Economy

Everyone who has ever run track has seen it—the inevitable tall lanky guy who reaches out as far in front of him as he can with his lead leg attempting to cover as much ground as he can with each stride. Everyone who has seen this guy run also knows he is usually not leading the pack.

Why is this guy covering so much ground with each stride, yet going so slow? It's because instead of using his forward inertia to push him ahead, he is slightly putting on the brakes by landing heal first. Every time he does this, he is fighting his inertia to go forward, thus slowing himself down as opposed to speeding up. Rather, bring your lead knee up high, close to your butt, to reduce torque and increase the distance covered with each stride; this will also lengthen your stride, and you will land with your center of mass slightly in front of your lead leg. Making initial contact with your heel is OK, but land at an angle allowing you to flow from the heel, to the midfoot, to the big toe without losing forward inertia.

Another big thing I see often with runners is once they hit the ground and push off, they forget that they must keep moving that leg. Once your foot hits the ground, it is not only important to push off but to do so as quickly as possible reducing your contact time on the ground and then bringing your foot up close to the glute rather than letting it hang down low and swing back to the front. By bringing your foot up so that your heel is close to the glute, it reduces the lever arm, thus making it easier to bring the foot back to the front and repeat the process. With time and proper training if you focus on using these key points, your running economy will improve significantly.

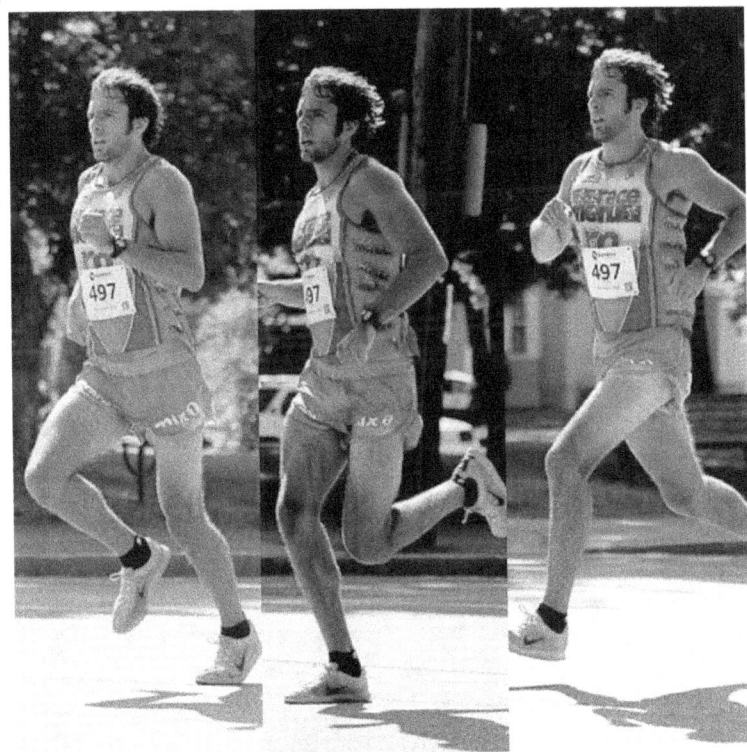

When most athletes hear the word "tension," what do you think is the first thing that comes to mind? Tight hamstrings, tendon sprains, and fascia tears? We all know more tension means more strain on the body, which can put it out of commission for weeks on end if not properly handled. But what about a little planned tension incorporated into your training? Our human movement system stores and releases energy like an elastic band, so wouldn't that make a little purposeful tension buildup good for athletic performance? Yes. Have you ever gone into competition after a proper taper (a planned reduction in training so you come back feeling refreshed) and felt sluggish and slow, even though you performed all the work exactly as planned up until your taper, at which point you cut back on your volume and reduced your intensity drastically (perhaps too drastically)? Think about it for a second, if low tension results in reduced energy production by your movement system; then it also means less force production and decreased quickness.

What does this mean to you? Next time you go to start your taper or have a competition coming up, use the following tips to keep tension high without over working. Keep duration short three days before the competition, asphalt rather than wood chips or soft dirt for running and plyometrics for ball sports. The extra tension may be just what you need to spring you toward a new personal record (PR).

Adequate Tension in Your Muscles Keeps Them Responsive

On the other hand, what if you are in the middle of building up your volume or intensity and you do not have a competition for a while? Is it safe to keep all that tension? No, having too much tension all the time is how athletes become injured. The key is to always have the right amount of tension. Sometimes you may need to lower tension, if that is the case, reduce speed work, plyometrics, and power training, shifting gears from a higher theme of PTS back to an earlier theme. Longer sessions will keep up your training volume, but the lower intensity will allow you to recover quicker between sessions, while allowing you to focus on proper movement patterns, which will result in less muscle-tissue breakdown. Try using these techniques during your training cycle so you can keep the right amount of tension always to help avoid injury and increase performance. The key is to maintain balance, use tension adding techniques when you haven't been competing or training hard and need to add some reactiveness and use tension reducing techniques when you have been racing or training hard and need to reduce some stress.

Reduce Speed Work, Plyometrics, and Power Training if You Become Lethargic

Quick, you're running away from an angry dog, bully, or bill collector and what's the first thing you do? Try and move your legs as fast as possible, right? The faster they go, the faster you go, right? Correct, the only problem is everyone moves their legs at roughly the same rate for a given speed. Peter Weyand performed a study on speed where he discovered that regardless of whether someone is a world class sprinter or an average Joe, The amount of time each stride takes is very similar (Weyand et al. 2000).

With this said, how do you increase your speed as well as your chances of a college scholarship or championship? Develop power throughout the whole body. Emphasize the lower extremities because they perform much of the work, but don't neglect the rest of your body. A well-rounded body is important because human movement is integrated (works as one unit). For the human movement system to work at its best, it needs to be a fine-tuned machine in its entirety.

To enhance strength (heavy power in PTS), perform exercises almost entirely at or above 85 percent of your one-repetition maximum, which is roughly equal to sets of five repetitions or less, while focusing on keeping good form. Eighty-five percent of your 1RM is the threshold that many strength development traits activate. Great examples of lower body lifts are your dead lifts, squats, and step ups.

Strength is Increased with Heavy Sets of Five Reps or Less

When it comes to increasing power (work over time), use plyometrics. Using a lighter load with very quick reaction (max power in PTS), as well as heavier loads that take slightly longer to execute. Examples are jump rope and depth jump to leap respectively. Once your feet are off the ground, regardless of who you are, you will have the same hang time while in the air (elites take less steps over the same distance due to launch, they don't stay in the air for a longer time, just cover more ground while in the air).

Plyometrics Help You Cover More Distance with Each Step

Did you know that by adding the same training techniques used by quick-reaction sports such as basketball, soccer, and lacrosse, distance runners can become better at distance running? It's true. This is due to a phenomenon known as the stretch-shortening cycle (SSC). The SSC is a progression that occurs to the muscles during movement. This progression takes the muscles from their relaxed state to a state of extreme tension where energy is stored like an elastic band and then released, just like when you release a spring gun and a foam dart fires.

Why is this progression important to your running career? Well, the less time your muscles are in that extreme state of tension, the lesser the energy lost. Therefore, by practicing plyometrics, you can decrease the time it takes you to go from storing energy to using energy, performing the act of running with more efficiency and less energy cost.

Think of it this way, when you run a race, you eventually slow down your cadence resulting in each foot strike lasting longer on the ground. By doing plyometrics, not only are you shortening the time wasted by your foot remaining in contact with the ground, but you are using "free" energy stored up in the muscles, tendons, ligaments, and fascia consequently saving energy for later in the race.

Additionally, plyometrics will help your body absorb the ground reaction forces (forces that the ground exerts on you as you push off the ground) by strengthening and preparing the connective tissue to better distribute that force. Now that you know this secret weapon, be sure to use it. But remember, plyometrics should not be used more than once or twice a week, and sparingly during the peak of your competitive season as competition is already demanding a lot from your body.

Now you know what you need to do to increase your speed, improve launch time by increasing launch force and decreasing contact time, "launch time." Again, do this by lifting heavy, performing plyometrics, and sprinting.

"Launch Time" is the Amount of Time Your Foot is in Contact with the Ground

Reactive strength is your body's ability to react as quickly as possible to a stimulus. If you think about it, that covers just about every moment in sports, catching a pass, covering the offense, or drafting off an opponent. Reactive strength also prepares you for real-life situations, catching something that is falling, catching yourself when falling, dodging something, tactical situations, or just keeping up with family and friends. How many times have you found yourself having to react quickly to an event during your everyday activities? I would assume often.

When it comes down to it, reactive strength is the premise behind not only sports but all of life. Life is random, and we must react to it, so why not be ready for the random? Although we cannot predict what is going to happen, we sure can cut down on reaction time, saving us during the big game.

Your Ability to React Quickly is Essential in all Sports

When training for reactive strength, it is best to utilize reaction exercises (big surprise, I know). Utilize reaction balls and partner directional drills. Get one of those little balls with all the bumps, toss it in the air, let it bounce, and then chase it. Or find a partner and perform depth jump to sprints or fire feet to acceleration drills in the direction your partner randomly points or shouts.

It is also important to be able to produce great amounts of power. Therefore, you should continue performing high-velocity exercises such as plyometrics and Olympic lifts along with heavy load exercises to keep up your strength.

Staying on top of your reactive strength is vital to your game. All the strength training in the world will not help your game if it takes you half an hour to react to a pass. Remember, athletes need to train like athletes, not school buses. That is quick and agile, not big, slow, annoying, and always in the way.

Athletics has a way of inspiring us to go longer, faster, and harder because we can see the result appear before our eyes. With athletics, you physically become the result of your efforts.

With that said, we can sometimes get carried away in our training and take it too far too often. Don't get me wrong, pushing yourself is the only way to get better. You must introduce your body to a new harder stimulus for it to adapt and improve. It is when you insert these hard efforts too often with too little break that trouble can start creeping up in the form of overtraining. Overtraining is the result of too much stimulus with too little time to adapt that causes a decrease in performance. The key is noticing the signs of overtraining and cutting back your training before it gets too late and your performance deteriorates.

Here are some common signs and symptoms of overtraining to look out for:

- Decrease in muscle mass
- Decrease in strength
- Decrease or disrupted sleep
- Depression
- Fatigue
- Increased resting heart rate
- Irritability
- Joint pain

If you are experiencing some of the descriptions above, you may be overtraining. If so then here are some things you can do to fix the problem:

- Stay active; decrease your training by lowering your volume, frequency, and/or intensity for one to two weeks. If this doesn't work, then you may need to take some time off completely.
- Participate in cross-training activities to reduce the stress on your muscles and joints commonly used during training.
- Relax your diet for a few days if it is typically very strict. Conversely, eat healthier if you normally eat foods with poor nutritional value.
- Relook at your diet, and make sure it is structured to your needs. A typical athlete's diet should be composed of 55–60 percent carbohydrates, 30 percent fat (10 percent or less of which is from saturated fat), and 10–15 percent protein.
- Switch up your routine completely. Upon returning to the gym after your break, engage in a routine with less structure for a while before getting serious again.

Overtraining Will Diminish Reactive Strength

Making a Box to Keep Your Spine Safe

Making a "box" while lifting is a fundamental yet often overlooked aspect of proper power- and weight-lifting form. Powerlifting involves the squat, bench press, and deadlift, generally performed slower while weightlifting revolves around the more explosive snatch and clean and jerk. The purpose of forming a box is to keep the spine safe while moving loads during variations of the deadlift as well as overhead movements. It is important to adopt making a box as part of your routine early on, so when weight increases, proper form is already embedded in your technique.

The first step in making a box is rolling your shoulders back and retracting your scapula (wing bones). A good indicator of this is your chest will stick out and your shoulders are low and behind your ears.

The second step is increasing intra-abdominal pressure. By increasing intra-abdominal pressure, low level activation for light loads, and bracing strategies for heavier loads, you are stabilizing your spine in preparation for the load (Osar, 2012). Transversus abdominis exercises such as vacuums and supine marching are excellent for intra-abdominal contraction strength. On a side note, these two exercises are also beneficial for avoiding and remedying abdominal separation triggered by pregnancy.

The third and final step is proper hip alignment in relation to your belly button and sternum (bottom of the rib cage). Your sternum, belly button, and hips should always line up. This will reduce back arching. Note: Sometimes people's belly button sticks out further than it should be (eat more greens and drink less alcohol); if this is the case, portray a flat abdomen's belly button placement when aligning your core.

There you have it, the proper way to make a box and keep your spine safe when lifting. Use this technique when lifting light loads, so it is instinctual when you progress to heavier loads.

1. Roll Shoulders Back
2. Increase Intra-Abdominal Pressure
3. Proper Hip Alignment

*Please see the pictures on the following pages for an example of how to properly make a box.

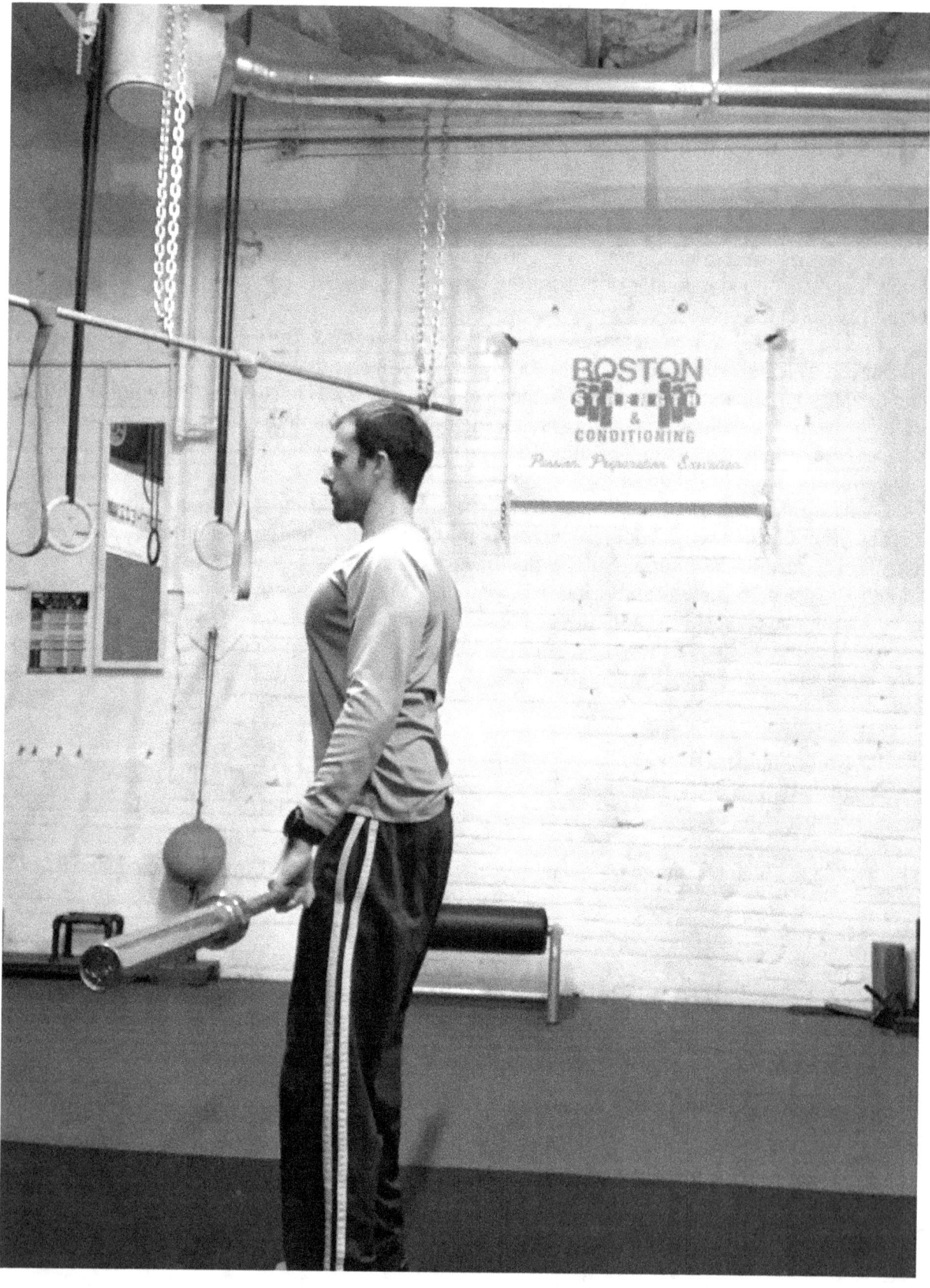

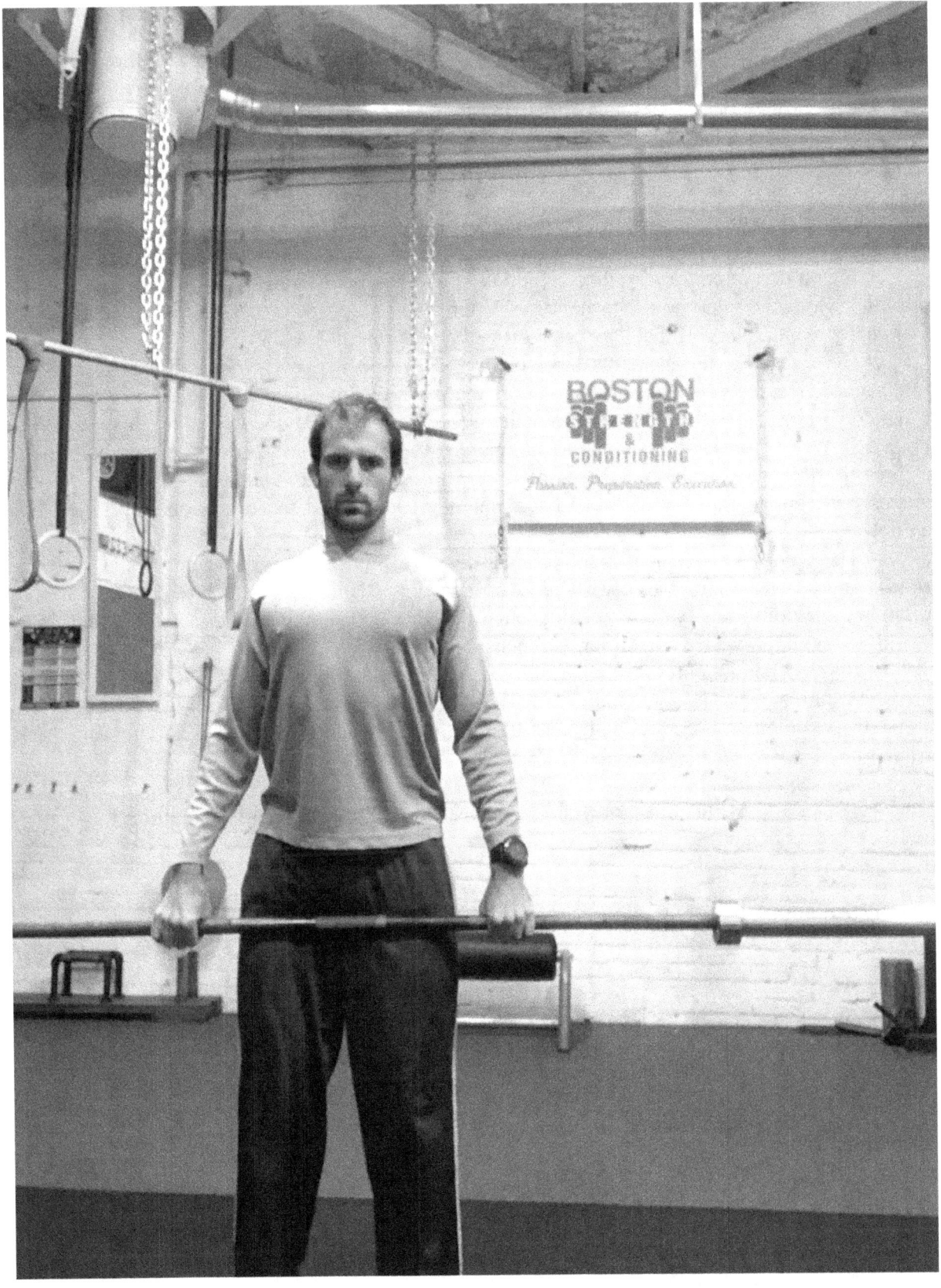

Even as a competitive distance runner, it boggles my mind seeing people who do nothing but run on the treadmill for their workouts. If you look at any competitive runner's routine, you will see a professionally designed cross-training resistance program going along with her running. "Well, I'm not a competitive runner; I just want to get in a quick workout and burn a lot of calories fast." Was that your answer? If all you do is run, then all you are doing is working the same few muscles repeatedly. Point being all this repetitiveness is going to lead to chronic overuse injuries if you are not working the opposing muscles that become imbalanced by strictly running and using the other muscles in your body that are being ignored.

If you do not perform well-rounded workouts that incorporate every major muscle group and only work the same joints in the same pattern without proper cross-training, then you will eventually get an injury. If that happens, you will not be running at all.

Here are two key elements I personally use in most of my cross-training. The first is multijoint movements. This means using more than one joint at a time during each exercise. How often do you just stand there and curl something (besides beer, that doesn't count; this is a fitness book). So why not make the move more natural and turn it into a suitcase row when you stand in a three-fourths squat position and row a barbell up like a suitcase. You are still performing a biceps curl, but you also work your back, shoulder, and the triple extension (hip, knee, and ankle).

The second key element is multiplanar or exercising in every direction: frontal (left and right), sagittal (front and back), vertically (up and down), and transversely (rotation and anti-rotation). By doing this, we are keeping our body in balance. We live in a three-dimensional world, so shouldn't we train in all three dimensions?

By incorporating cross-training into your routine, regardless of sport, your body becomes prone to fatigue and injury, leading to a more successful career. Even if you are not a competitive athlete, no one wants to miss training or performing fun activities with family and friends.

Multijoint-Multiplanar Exercises Improve Overall Mechanics

Time Under Tension: Training by Time

Unless we are taught how to properly vary our workouts, we all go to the gym and perform eight to twelve reps per set with a sixty-second rest between every set. We do this week after week expecting change, yet we are not exposing ourselves to enough variation for our body to adapt to something new. We need to change the way we train if we expect our body to change. With that said, have any of you ever tried training by time?

Rather than trying to hit a set number of repetitions, aim for a set amount of time keeping the muscle under constant tension for that period. This is a great way to change up your workout for two reasons.

First, since physiological adaptations occur based on time under tension and not reps, we can more clearly pinpoint when we are transferring to a different energy system (they all contribute at one time, but one system is always more dominant). Additionally, muscle fiber recruitment is enhanced by increasing the frequency of activation (the longer the muscle is stressed, the more fibers are engaged). Training by time does not force us to put on the brakes when we get to a certain rep but rather forces us to go until we are done.

There are different energy systems based on your training goal. In a nutshell, our phosphagen system quickly supplies us with energy that last for up to ten seconds. After that energy is depleted, we shift to the glycolysis phase, which uses glucose (sugar in our bloodstream) as energy. This energy system can supply us for roughly two minutes. At this point the oxidative system is ready to kick in, and we switch from anaerobic exercise to aerobic exercise using more fats as our primary resource.

Phosphagen = <10 s; Glycolysis = 2 min; Oxidative = >2 min

Nowhere in that description did I mention any energy system being measured by repetitions! It was all measured by time. Doesn't it make sense to train by time? If we understand the proper intensities for each period and the adaptations that occur by training in that time frame, our results will be more precise toward our goal than training by repetitions.

Here is an example for hypertrophy muscle building by time:

Twenty to sixty seconds at 75–85 percent intensity with a work-to-rest ratio of 1:1 lasting for a total of fifteen to twenty minutes per muscle group.

Another great breakdown for power training is the following:

Five to ten seconds at 90–100 percent intensity with a work-to-rest ratio of 1:6–1:12 lasting for fifteen to twenty minutes per muscle group.

Next time you're resistance training, try one of these formulas, and see if you feel the difference after your first session.

Everything that was ever invented has a purpose, otherwise it would never have been thought up. Nonetheless, that does not mean the purpose had a positive effect. With that said, machines in fitness centers are a prime example of good intent with a poor outcome. Granted, machines do have their place in rehabilitation settings for reactivating the underactive muscle prior to reintegrating it into functional movements or rebalancing muscular imbalances. Other than that, they are counterproductive.

Fitness resistance machines were well adopted by novices lacking proper guidance when beginning a mechanical training program as well as the bodybuilding community aiming to overload specific muscles, mainly the prime movers, paying less attention to stabilizing muscles. Knowing this, resistance machines have introduced people into weight rooms who otherwise may be intimidated, which is good, but a better approach would be if weight rooms took a few minutes to explain the value of free weights over machines as well as how to properly use free weights.

Think about it. The order in which training is progressed is from stability to strength and then to power exercises. So why are we starting off with loads we cannot handle freely but rather stabilized by a machine? If we are to follow the correct method of progression, we should learn to stabilize the free weight prior to loading up the muscle (see *The PROformance Training Systems Progression Model*).

Also, machines allow us to overload the muscle during its initial contraction while it's at its furthest point of extension, leading to unnecessary and even harmful load during the initial contraction that may lead to muscle or tendon damage. In extreme cases a tear can occur. Moreover, muscles have four main jobs: motion, maintain posture, protection, and produce heat. If exercise is an attempt at making people more efficient at the motions/task, then why are we using a machine that works our muscles in isolated contractions? Think about it, this is the exact opposite of why we are here in the first place. And if muscles are also supposed to maintain posture, then why are we using machines to simulate movement in the most stable plane possible? Shouldn't we be exercising in unstable environments if we are trying to adapt to the demands of everyday life and sport? Remember the Sea Squirt? I feel resistance machines provoke the Sea Squirt mentality during exercise. Wasting the gift of movement. Strength transfers from unstable environments to stable ones but not as significantly the other way around, so work your way up to an environment as unstable as your lifestyle entails.

Training in Unstable Positions Improves Stable Performance but Not Vice Versa

Somewhere over the past few decades, resistance machine use during exercise received public support from people in the fitness industry; that pull has caused a lot of injuries and slowly progressing athletes. I say it is time to dump the machines and utilize free weights. Start off light and simple, and work your way up. I'm not saying to go out there and start performing a clean and jerk on your first day. I'm saying perform a dumbbell press as opposed to a machine chest press. I guarantee you'll feel the difference after your first set. You'll hear your body saying, "Thanks for finally training me the way you want me to perform."

Don't Train Like a Sea Squirt

During every step we take, cutting maneuver we make, or jump we land, we are placing extreme levels of force on our muscles, tendons, and ligaments. During every action we perform, gravity is constantly pulling us downward resulting in a continuous eccentric demand that our bodies must meet.

Additionally, as gravity is pulling us down, the ground is pushing back against us. This is known as ground reaction force. Moreover, as our velocity and amplitude increase, so do the ground reaction forces our body encounters.

For that reason, our bodies are consistently undergoing eccentric demands. Yet the primary objective many of us focus on while training for athletic competition is concentric movement (accelerating our bodies or objects) not eccentric movement (decelerating our body or objects).

This focus of training results in injury. It is not the motions that our bodies are trained for that cause injury but the ones that we are ill-prepared for that result in a tear, sprain, or break.

Very rarely does someone injure something mid-workout unless he is excessively tight or their pre-practice hydration levels are not balanced. It is during a breaking movement (stopping, cutting, landing) that injury results. And yes, injury does occur during acceleration too, which is a result of lack of conditioning emphasis on acceleration and too much emphasis on max speed. We accelerate and are forced to stop prior to reaching max speed more frequently than we are cruising along down the field full throttle, so why not focus more on deceleration? It's clear that eccentric action training should receive as much if not more emphasis during conditioning than concentric training.

Deceleration Training Is Essential for Injury Prevention

Remodel your workout, taking this knowledge into account. Rather than focusing all your energy of the lift portion of the movement you are performing, focus on the lowering portion. Try taking four seconds to lower the object you are moving during every rep of your next workout, and you will feel the difference the next morning when you wake up. Additionally, spend more time on deceleration drills when practicing movement drills on the field or court. Lack of attention to these drills along with rotational drills during practice is why athletes are injury prone during competition.

And now the other side of the coin, I remember growing up watching coaches of speed and power sports (baseball, football, etc.) send their athletes out on long runs for training. What I always wondered when I saw this was when do baseball players run long distances during a game? The answer is never. Although long runs can help athletes with weight control in the off season, and I recommend shorter base building running lasting up to twenty minutes in the early stages of the off-season to improve aerobic capacity and raise the ventilatory threshold without the repetitive pounding of sprints, there are much more sports-specific ways to train ball based sports.

Hear me out. If a high-school basketball court is twenty-eight yards, what's an eight-mile run going to do for your athletes? Nothing. Yes, of course, it will increase their VO_2max and fat efficiency but so will long-sprint intervals. And the higher intensity of those intervals is much more sport specific than that of an eight-mile run.

HIIT is More Beneficial Than a Long Run for Ball Sports

Let's go a little deeper, how often do any of these athletes sprint for more than thirty meters? Very rarely, if ever. That is why emphasis of speed training should be on acceleration drills. All-out sprints that are no longer than twenty to thirty meters should be a primary goal of conditioning sessions. A great example of one of these workouts is twenty meters all-out sprint with a work-to-rest interval of 1:6 or ten-second hill sprints with a work-to-rest interval of 1:6. By training in this manner, you are focusing on the energy system used during competition.

All right, now we understand why it is so important to perform acceleration drills. Let's get into the biomechanics of it all. Picture a world class 100-meter sprinter. When she gets out of the blocks, she is leaning forward driving her feet into the ground while pumping her arms like crazy, right? The same goes for any other sport involving linear acceleration. Lean forward to carry your inertia and enhance your arm cadence to initiate forward drive.

With that said, let's examine the difference in muscle usage from a long-run to acceleration. During a distance run, the main muscles used are the hamstrings and hip flexors to keep the body in motion. Conversely, while accelerating, there is more use by the quadriceps and glutes as they drive your feet into the ground propelling your body to maximum velocity as quickly as possible. Therefore, it is important to incorporate squats and step ups into the athletes training regime when focusing on enhancing acceleration.

This and the last chapter bring up a valuable point. In science, you can almost always find research supporting two viewpoints. The ability to understand the difference and potential values of both is where experience plays a role. Look for validity and reliability in the research you read, and remember, sometimes scientist prove what coaches already know. Just as every story has two sides, sometimes science can as well.

Compound versus Isolation Exercises

While at the gym, if you stop and look around for a minute you're going to see two types of people: people who exercise using compound movements and people who exercise using isolated movements. Although in an ideal world people will be using a combination of both to ensure their body is getting the well-rounded attention it needs to work optimally; realistically most people do not know better. But that is OK, because you do! Isolated exercises are exercises working strictly on one muscle area such as a leg curl focusing primarily on the hamstring or triceps pushdown for the triceps. These types of exercises work at one joint only with emphasis strictly on the muscles moving that joint. Working in this manner allows for "attention to detail" for the muscle if there is an imbalance. The most useful time for isolation exercises is during rehabilitation or corrective exercise when rebalancing weak and tight or elongated and taut muscles is the focus.

Compound or multijoint exercises are just that, exercises working multiple joints at the same time. Examples of these are the squat for the glutes, quads, and hamstrings or bench press for the chest, shoulders, and triceps. Lifting this way accomplishes a couple of things. First, it is the primary method of attaining overall muscle-mass gains; second, it is the way our body moves in everyday life or functional training as it is commonly referred. As mentioned earlier, unless there is a muscle imbalance or area prone to muscle imbalance, compound exercises are typically the way to go.

Compound Exercises Increase Strength Quicker than Isolation Exercises

Understanding Repetition Ranges and Rest Intervals

I want to talk about the importance of proper repetition ranges and rest intervals for resistance training, how they vary between workout goals, and what those ranges and intervals are.

Training Objectives by Repetition Range

Objective (Goal) of Training	Repetitions
Muscular Endurance	15–20+
Hypertrophy (Size)	8–12
Strength	4–8
Power	1–4(Heavy) or 6–10 (Fast & Light)

Power

Strength

Hypertrophy (Size)

Muscular Endurance

Every workout serves a different purpose; some are for power or strength and others for endurance. So why would every workout have the same repetition range and rest interval between sets? Think about it, why would you have a long rest and low repetition range if you are working on muscular endurance? Since we are trying to condition our body to resist fatigue, we should not give it long periods of time to recover; we should give it high-volume workloads with short rest. Vice versa, if the objective is to increase power, we cannot generate max or near maximum power if we are tired from too little rest and doing high volume with low-weight sets.

Goal of Training	Time
Muscular Endurance	10–30 sec.
Hypertrophy (Size)	30–90 sec.
Strength	2–3 min. (120–180 sec.)
Power	3–5 min. (180–300 sec.)

Power

Strength

Hypertrophy (Size)

Muscular Endurance

These ranges match up with a certain amount of muscle recruitment type and ratio. When you start changing the ranges, you start changing the workout.

Now that you have a clearer picture of why it is important to track how long each rest period is and why they are valuable, let's look at the duration of rest intervals.

In general, the above chart lists the most commonly agreed upon rest intervals for each type of workout. Start paying attention to these rest intervals and their corresponding repetition ranges, and you will undoubtedly see an increase in performance in just a few weeks. Violate the rest rules, and you will lose focus on your training objectives primary goal and slow your progress toward optimal performance.

It can become complicated understanding when to employ HIIT training. HIIT focuses on combining a variety of training goals, and because of this you, will experience a variety of less than optimal progress in each area being trained. However, this is not a bad thing and HIIT does have its place in sports training. During competition for most ball sports, you are competing in a manner very similar to HIIT. Athletes on the field or court are constantly accelerating and decelerating, maneuvering, jumping, reaching, and twisting at a wide range of intensities for varying periods of time. Most sports do not focus on exceeding in any single discipline, but rather the correct combination of attributes to execute all the moves of the sport. This makes HIIT sport specific to ball sports and thus should be included during the potential theme of PTS.

When you are resistance training, how many sets do you perform? Better yet, how many reps are you doing—2 × 15, 3 × 10, 4 × 6? Although there are specific ranges for results, there is no set-in stone range for everyone. What matters is how you perform those sets.

Whenever you are lifting for any training goal except corrective, it is essential that the last couple of reps in each set bring your working muscles to failure. It is during these final reps that you achieve gains, not during the first eight in a set of ten but in the last two. During that struggle to move the weight as you feel gravity slowly winning the battle is when you are causing the micro tears necessary to obtain the desired strength gains. According to Dr. Stephen Ball, PhD, 70 percent of strength gains are estimated to happen during the first set when performed to failure (Ball 2016).

70% of Strength Gains Happen During the First Set

While training, you need to reach failure to become successful. You will not get where you want unless you are continuously failing along the way. This principle not only applies to lifting but every form of exercise. Push yourself, adapt, push yourself some more. The key to lifting the correct amount of weight when lifting to failure is following the correct rest intervals from the previous chapter.

The "secret" is being willing to fail. Know that failure is pivotal to getting where you want to be. Don't be afraid to grunt a little in the gym or make a strange face because the weight is heavy. It's supposed to be that way. Remember, it is a gym, not a runway. Regardless of how many people appear to be there solely to take selfies. It's not supposed to be pretty. It's OK to let people know you're doing a little work; hopefully, they will see your ethic and jump on the band wagon. Set the example; be your gym's number one failure!

With that said, remember quality movement is much more important than the quantity of weight. You don't want to be the star of someone's fitness blooper meme of gif because you are swinging the bar wildly like a mad-man while doing curls in the squat rack. When moving these loads, be certain you are going through the full range of motion and could properly stabilize yourself and maintain good dynamic posture throughout the exercise. If you cannot move the weight with proper form, reduce the weight and build up to it for a future workout. And on a side note, please don't do curls in the squat rack.

Metabolic Training

High-Intensity Versus Low-Intensity Training

Cardiorespiratory fitness is a component of fitness concerned with aerobic capacity, VO_2max, and aerobic efficiency. Cardiorespiratory fitness improves with training the cardiovascular system and respiratory system. The cardiovascular system involves the transport of blood, nutrients, hormones, oxygen, and carbon dioxide throughout the body. It is governed by the cardiac output of the heart and utilizes arteries, veins, and capillaries for systemic transport of nutrients and removal of waste products (Baechle and Earle 2000, 119).

The respiratory system, which is also known as the ventilator system, is responsible for the exchange of gases throughout the body. By engaging the larynx, trachea, bronchi, lungs, and pleura along with the use of the cardiovascular system, the respiratory system is able the manage the oxygen and carbon dioxide exchange throughout the body and keep it in homeostasis regardless of its physical endeavors (Roberts 2000, 1). A proper exercise protocol focused on cardiorespiratory fitness empowers athletes to improve these factors increasing health and athletic performance.

As people attempt to pack more activities into their lives with no change in the time available to accomplish these activities, people have taken a liking into shorter and more intense forms of exercise. Here we will investigate if high-intensity training involving high levels of intensity over a shorter duration is as effective or more effective as long-duration exercise performed at a lower intensity. We will then examine similar research surrounding sprint training versus traditional endurance training comparing the adaptions and implications of the two exercise modes. Finally, a look at the relationship between walking and running economy will be compared. But first, a review of excess post-exercise oxygen consumption will be discussed to provoke initial thought on the different effects the two training modalities (high-intensity versus low-intensity training) have on the body.

Before investigating the difference between high-intensity interval training (HIIT) and prolonged lower-intensity training, a brief examination of excess post-exercise oxygen consumption (EPOC) is of significance because the nature of EPOC is an acute and clear indicator of the difference between high-intensity interval training and lower-intensity methods. Elevated respiration levels occurring during EPOC are the body's attempt to get back to homeostasis. Elevated respiration is clearly evidence during exercise and is a prime indicator that the individual is stressing his body.

Heavy Breathing Upon Completing an Interval is Known as EPOC

Gaesser and Brooks (1984) tackle the question why is there post-exercise oxygen consumption following physical activity. Gaesser and Brooks examine past research to answer this question. Gaesser and Brooks's research highlight a variety of explanations for post-exercise oxygen consumption. The first theory the researchers came across was performed in 1920 by Hill and his associates and states that O_2 debt is the result of the oxidation of a minor fraction (one-fifth) of the lactate formed during exercise, to provide the energy to reconvert the remainder (four-fifths) of the lactate to glycogen during recovery. Gasser and Brooks also examine more recent research by Margaria and their peers, building upon Hill's work by differentiating between initial, fast "alactacid," and second, slow "lactacid," O_2-debt curve components. Margaria and colleagues hypothesized that the fast phase of the post-exercise O_2-consumption curve was due to the restoration of phosphagen (ATP + CP). Numerous other studies were examined demonstrating a dissociation between the kinetics of lactate removal and the slow component of the post-exercise VO₂ in several species. Gasser and Brooks concluded their research by determining that no complete explanation of the post-exercise metabolism exists. However, there is a link between elevated post-exercise VO₂ and mitochondrial O₂ consumption for energy production. Moreover, elevated temperature is perhaps the most significant metabolic basis during this process. Since no explanation of EPOC exist, further research can consider training modalities reducing excess post-exercise oxygen consumption. This may shine light into the mechanisms involved in post-exercise oxygen consumption and how they relate to both high-intensity interval training and low-intensity training. By being aware of EPOC, there is acknowledgment that metabolic adaptions are occurring because of the training methodology. Regardless if it is high-intensity interval training or prolonged, traditional endurance training.

Several articles regarding high-intensity training aim at determining the skeletal and metabolic differences and potential benefits of high-intensity interval training versus traditional exercise (Gibala 2009; Little et al. 2010; Nybo et al. 2010). The research examines responses to fitness parameters such as VO₂max, resting heart rate, fat percentage, and lean mass as well as mitochondrial biogenesis variations between the two training methods and molecular responses to high-intensity interval training. Overall, findings suggest benefits both in response to exercise and duration necessary to gain these benefits from high-intensity interval training over traditional exercise.

HIIT is an Effective and Efficient Alternative to Traditional Exercise

A collection of articles regarding short-term sprint-interval training versus traditional endurance training investigates key differentiators between the two training methods. As with high-intensity interval training, sprint intervals are examined to determine if a training modality of higher intensity and shorter duration will have similar or greater benefits when compared with traditional endurance training considering the time-efficiency of sprint training (Burgomaster, Heigenhauser, and Gibala 2006; Burgomaster et al. 2008; Burgomaster et al. 2005; Gibala et al. 2006; Ross and Leveritt 2001). The researchers studied sprint interval training under a variety of circumstances, yet all conclude sprint training is a time-efficient method to increase skeletal muscle capacity and promote metabolic adaptions like that of traditional endurance training. However, I must highlight that sprint interval training should not be conducted without first developing adequate levels of mechanical control through strength training and metabolic capacity during the learn and prepare phases of PTS. If these preparatory steps are not taken, injury is more likely to occur.

Although the above research showcases profound evidence for high-intensity training over traditional methods, high-intensity training is not always possible for people for a variety of reasons ranging from heart disease, to injury, and to age. With that said, switching focus from high-intensity training modalities to walking investigates options for those who cannot participate in high-intensity interval training. Numerous studies examine walking's benefits (Duncan et al. 2005; Sawyer et al. 2010; Williams and Thompson 2013). However, the methods used vary between comparisons of walking and running as well as walking at four different exercise conditions. Due to the distinct nature of the studies, a direct comparison is difficult to make; however, all the studies reviewed did determine walking as a beneficial exercise-training modality compared to baseline.

The results of high-intensity interval training versus traditional exercise literature suggest practical uses for high-intensity interval training based on its findings. Research on molecular responses to high-intensity interval exercise found that high-intensity "induced rapid phenotypic changes that resemble traditional endurance training—the metabolic changes induced by high-intensity training, inducing mitochondrial biogenesis and an increased capacity for Glucose and fatty acid oxidation" (Gibala 2009). Additional research by Little and colleagues (2010) discovered after two weeks of six low-volume, high-intensity training sessions consisting of eight-to-twelve-by-sixty-second intervals at approximately 100 percent of peak power output showed an increase in exercise capacity as well as other metabolic variables associated with improving exercise performance. A third study by Nybo et al. (2010) examining high-intensity training versus traditional exercise interventions (prolonged running and strength training performed separately) for promoting health discovered benefits for both high-intensity training and traditional exercise methods. High-intensity training improved cardiorespiratory fitness (VO_2max) and glucose tolerance beyond that of traditional exercise interventions. However, prolonged running showed lower resting heart rate, lower fat percentage, and lower total and HDL plasma cholesterol than high-intensity training. Furthermore, strength training showed an increase in both bone mass and lean mass that high-intensity training did not provide.

Research Shows HIIT to be an Effective Substitute for Traditional Exercise

The results of the sprint interval training interventions are intriguing considering all the studies examined are looking at different variables. Yet all the studies are in favor of sprint training over traditional endurance training. Burgomaster, Heigenhauser, and Gibala (2006) examined the effects of short-term sprint interval training on skeletal-muscle glycogenolysis and lactate accumulation as well as an increase in the capacity for pyruvate oxidation via pyruvate dehydrogenase. Burgomaster and colleagues' results showed that two weeks consisting of six sessions of sprint interval training on eight men improve the three variables examined, leading to improved cycling time trial performance. Furthermore, a similar study by Burgomaster et al. (2006) found comparable findings concerning sprint interval training's effect on cycling ability. Burgomaster et al. found approximately fifteen minutes of intense sprint exercise over a two-week period increased muscle oxidative potential as well as endurance capacity in recreationally active people.

As Little as Two Weeks of Sprint Training Can Improve Endurance Capacity

Work by Burgomaster et al. (2008) discovered the metabolic adaptions during exercise after low-volume sprint interval training were like that of traditional endurance training. After six weeks of sprint interval training or traditional endurance training, participants (five men and five women per group) showed similar differences in mitochondrial markers for skeletal muscle carbohydrate and lipid metabolism as well as metabolic control given large variation in training volume and time commitment between the two training methods. Additional findings by Gibala and colleagues (2006) discovered that under similar training parameters but for a shorter duration (two weeks), skeletal muscle and exercise performance adaptions are comparable to endurance training in young active men regardless of the significant reduction in training duration and time involved in short-term sprint interval training. This reduction in time necessary to elicit the desired result allows for athletes to reduce overall training time and/or focus on additional PTS themes.

Sprint Training Maintains Progress, While Saving Time

A study by Ross and Leveritt (2001) investigates the long-term metabolic and skeletal muscle adaptions to short-sprint training, and their findings suggest the adaptions of sprint training vary depending on the variables of sprint training such as duration, frequency, amount, and rest of the sprint as well as individual differences among athletes. Enzyme adaptions as well as skeletal adaptions are all dependent on the individual sprinting, the sprinting parameters implemented, as well as the individual's response to that unique combination.

Sprinting Adaptions Vary Depending on Exercise Prescription

The findings of several articles on walking suggest walking as a beneficial means of exercise for maintaining health. Articles by Williams and Thompson (2013) found when moderate walking is compared with vigorous running, similar risk reductions for hypertension, hypercholesterolemia, diabetes mellitus, and potentially coronary heart disease were found when energy expenditure was the same. These findings are like Duncan et al. (2005) discovery that hard-intensity-low-frequency walking and moderate-intensity-high-frequency walking both provide improvements in cardiorespiratory fitness. Although walking was shown to produce similar health benefits to running, Sawyer et al. (2010) learned there is an inverse relationship between cardiorespiratory fitness and exercise economy as walking speed increases, meaning running is generally a smoother and more efficient movement than power walking. If VO_2peak is low and movement economy is high, resulting in an efficient gait, the same results can be attained as if they had a high VO_2peak and poor form. These findings are interesting and are worth further research to determine if this inverse relationship between cardiorespiratory fitness and exercise economy stands true as individuals' transition to running.

Walking is a Valuable Substitute for Athletes Who Cannot Run

After examining the above results comparing high-intensity interval training versus traditional endurance training and strength training (Gibala 2009; Little et al. 2010; Nybo et al. 2010), there is solid evidence that as little as two weeks of high-intensity interval training can produce similar adaptions to traditional endurance training. However, the research methods used compared sprint-cycling to endurance-cycling methods and sprint-running to endurance-running methods. An interesting study would be to compare high-intensity interval training composed of exercises such as burpees, mountain climbers, and battle ropes against high-intensity sprint-cycling intervals, sprint-running intervals, and strength training. Although these exercise modalities are drastically different, they are all meant to serve a similar purpose (improve cardiorespiratory fitness and strength). Therefore, blood samples and muscles biopsies comparing metabolic and strength adaptions would be of interest to determine which method produces the greatest physical adaption and the most effective weekly time commitment.

The articles concerning sprint training represent a more focused version of the articles about high-intensity interval training (Burgomaster, Heigenhauser, and Gibala 2006; Burgomaster et al. 2008; Burgomaster et al. 2005; Gibala et al. 2006; Ross and Leveritt 2001).

The results of the sprint interval-training research all suggest that although there is significantly lower time commitment associated with sprint training when compared with traditional endurance training, similar adaptions are present. The question is would the benefits have a compound effect if sprint-training was paired with traditional endurance exercise? The research compares the two training methods, but what if a third group was studied comparing concurrent sprint and traditional endurance exercise versus sprint-training versus traditional endurance exercise? Would the combined group outperform the two singular training-method groups? Furthermore, the studies focused on a single-interval duration of sprint intervals for each given study. What if a study compared traditional endurance training versus a mixed-interval-duration sprint session (e.g., one set at 10 s, 30 s, 60 s, 75 s, 90 s, and 120 s), then what would the findings of a test formatted in this manner suggest? Questions such as these allow for further research. This is why coaching with all the recent advances in science is still an art.

Walking is Effective for Populations That Should Avoid High Stress Training

In closing, society has refined American culture focusing on time efficiency as well as maximizing value within that given time. With that said, medicine, science, and technology are collaborating to bring attention to America's growing health concerns. With medicine and science discovering what needs to be done to improve American health and technology implementing new techniques of engaging people to improve their health. This hybrid between fields is the perfect opportunity to convince busy people to begin implementing relatively non-time-consuming exercise programs such as the ones justified in the above research into their lives, prolonging life as well as increasing its quality.

Athletes Should Use New Technologies to Monitor Their Health

Cardiorespiratory fitness is another way of describing someone's aerobic capacity or ability to do aerobic work. Numerous studies have shown that cardiorespiratory fitness is highly positively correlated with health and mortality. This chapter reviews a selection of research concerning cardiorespiratory fitness's link with health and mortality. The first review by Farrell, Fitzgerald, McAuley, and Barlow (2010) examines cardiorespiratory fitness's association with adiposity and all-cause mortality in women. The research involved 11,335 women who completed a comprehensive baseline examination between 1970 and 2005. The researchers used body mass index (BMI), waist circumference (WC), waist-to-height ratio (W/HT), waist-to-hip ratio (W/Hip), percent body fat (%BF), and CRF quantified as duration of a maximal exercise test as their clinical measures for examination. Years later, follow-up measures were taken, and it was observed that heart rate for all-cause mortality were lower as cardiorespiratory fitness increased. Adjusted death rates of overweight/obese women within each adiposity exposure were higher compared with normal-weight women and approached statistical significance for BMI, %BF, and W/HT. Heart rate were significantly higher in unfit women within each stratum of BMI compared with fit–normal BMI women. Fit women with high %BF had no greater risk of death compared with fit–normal-weight women. This shows lower cardiorespiratory fitness is positively correlated and thus a good indicator of all-cause mortality in women. Applications for these results are promoting role models for healthier images of woman in media focusing on aerobic capacity over poor dieting/fad diet habits that are typically found in media outlets (Van Vonderen and Kinnally 2012).

A similar study was performed by Farrell, Cortese, LaMonte, and Blair (2007) regarding cardiorespiratory fitness, different measures of adiposity, and mortality in men. The study was composed of 38,410 apparently healthy men completing a compressive baseline health examination between 1970 and 2001. Clinical measures of the exam included BMI, waist circumference (WC), percent body fat, and CRF quantified as duration of a maximal treadmill-exercise test. The participants were divided into five different stratums for each measurement. When grouped into categories of fit and unfit, mortality rates were significantly lower in fit compared with unfit men within each stratum of BMI, WC, and percent body fat. These findings reveal that higher levels of cardiorespiratory fitness are associated with lower risk of cancer mortality in men. To apply this study to medicine. Farrell et al.'s results should be shared with all families who have known cancer risk. In hopes of educating high cancer-risk individuals about the importance of cardiorespiratory fitness for lowering their risk of cancer.

Being Fit Reduces Mortality and Cancer Risk

Furthermore, heart disease is the leading cause of death for men, claiming one in four lives (CDC 2013). It is important to implement strength-training protocols in all men's lifestyles (as well as women for that matter). Research by Roberts, Katiraie, Croymans, Yang, and Kelesidis (2013) uncovered that young untrained men have dysfunctional HDL compared to strength-trained men. This was independent of weight. With the potential of saving one in four lives, strength training should be a mandatory component of all young men's educational curriculum. Roberts et al. research proves strength training may be one of the most important lessons a young man can learn concerning health.

With the Potential to Save 1 in 4 Lives, Learning How to Strength Train is Invaluable

Another study regarding cardiorespiratory fitness and mortality was performed on older adults. The research by Sui, LaMonte, Laditka, Hardin, Chase, Hooker, and Blair (2007) was investigating if cardiorespiratory fitness and adiposity can be used as a predictor of mortality in older adults. The study consisted of 2,603 adults aged sixty or older enrolled in the Aerobics Center Longitudinal Study who completed a baseline health examination during 1979–2001. A maximal exercise test was imposed to rank fitness and body mass index (BMI), waist circumference, and percent body fat used to measure adiposity. The researchers concluded fitness as a predictor of mortality risk in older adults independent of overall and abdominal adiposity. As a result, medical and health practitioners should recommend regular physical activity among older adults.

We All Need More Health Education to Reduced Mortality

Franklin (2009) understood regular physical activity is important for cardiovascular health. As a result, Franklin set out to see if there is a connection between exercise capacity and future health outcomes. What Franklin discovered is a high level of cardiorespiratory fitness (aerobic capacity) markedly reduces one's risk of cardiovascular disease, and the reduction is greater compared with merely being physically active. Franklin also discovered an inverse relationship between cardiorespiratory fitness and complications after bariatric surgery among morbidly obese adults. As well as an inverse relationship with health care cost. These correlations signify exercise capacity can indeed work as a crystal ball when it comes to certain health concerns.

Increases in Cardiovascular Health are Related to Decreases in Healthcare Cost

Discoveries such as Franklin's highlight the importance of fitness in health settings. Gregory Degnan, MD, is a believer and advocate for integration of fitness professionals into the healthcare continuum. Although Dr. Degnan believes fitness professionals need to overcome their stereotype as "ex jocks" by increasing their training, education, and certifications if they want to be taken more seriously in healthcare. With that said, Dr. Degnan believes and I concur, bringing fitness and healthcare professionals together is the ultimate step in preventative care (Bryant 2014, 76–77).

Fitness and Health Care Professionals Need to Work Together

The above reviews clearly show the benefits of cardiorespiratory fitness for overall health and mortality. Evidence shows that physical activity exercise capacity and cardiorespiratory capacity was shown to improve quality of life. With this said, the American College of Sports Medicine's recommendation of at least 150 minutes of moderate-intensity exercise per week for adults, which can be met through thirty to sixty minutes of moderate-intensity exercise (five days per week) or twenty to sixty minutes of vigorous-intensity exercise (three days per week) should be strictly followed (ACSM 2014).

ACSM Recommends at Least 150 Minutes of Moderate-Intensity Exercise Per Week

Moving beyond general health into athletic performance, the cardiorespiratory system has tremendous impact on athletic ability affecting metabolic mechanisms such as lactic acid, lactate, and VO_2max. More on the cardiorespiratory system's role in sports performance will be covered in the following chapters. If athletes understand how these metabolic mechanisms are affected by training, they can better customize their training to support optimal sport performance.

Looking back at the above research, cardiorespiratory physiology plays a major role from quality and length of life to athletic performance. Recent advances in science allow medical professionals to use exercise capacity as a predictor of mortality (Franklin 2009). As well as give fitness practitioners the knowledge to manipulate fitness training protocols to elicit specific metabolic responses to achieve a desired physical ability from their athletes.

Vitals Sharing is a Valuable Link Between Fitness and Medical Professionals

Moreover, an abundant amount of research has been published indicating that fitness training's effects on cardiorespiratory physiology is a necessity of life. Without fitness training quality and length of life diminishes. Therefore, appropriate steps in health policy should be taken to promote fitness throughout communities by educating students in schools, patients in hospitals, and older persons through community outreach events. Medical and health professionals need to have a fond understanding of fitness training or a reliable source they can send their patients to for learning and coaching them through active and healthy fitness lifestyles.

Medical and Health Professionals Should Have an Understanding of Fitness Training

Exercise physiology is the study of acute and chronic adaptions of the body to exercise. Traditionally exercise physiology has examined the effects of exercise in clinical settings affecting rehabilitation patients, but recently more resources have been spent on exercise's effects on athletes. The American Society of Exercise Physiologist (2014) best describes exercise physiology as:

> The identification of physiological mechanisms underlying physical activity and regular exercise, the comprehensive delivery of treatment services concerned with the analysis, improvement, and maintenance of physical and mental health and fitness, the rehabilitation of heart disease and other diseases and/or disabilities, and the professional guidance and counsel of athletes and others interested in athletics and sports training. (para. 2)

With this said, research and understanding of exercise physiology as well as experienced and knowledgeable practitioners of exercise physiology are essential for progress in exercise and sport. The following examines previous and current literature regarding an array of nutritional and exercise-induced effects pertaining to exercise physiology and what these findings represent for the field of exercise physiology and their implications to performance.

With a steadily increasing obesity epidemic, interest in fat metabolism has been growing over the past thirty years. Jeukendrip, Saris, and Wagenmakers (1998a) investigated deeply into fat mobilization and metabolism in their research, "Fat Metabolism during Exercise: A review—Part I: Fatty Acid Mobilization and Muscle Metabolism." The review covers lipolysis and its function in allowing fatty acids to enter the bloodstream. From the bloodstream, these fatty acids find their way into muscles and cross the mitochondrial membrane in muscle through the carnitine palmitoyltransferase system where the acyl CoA is degraded to acetyl CoA for oxidation in the citric acid cycle. In other words, how we use fat as fuel.

During the study of Jeukendrip, Saris, and Wagenmakers (1998),the team of researchers went on to discuss the two limiting factors of fatty-acid mobilization and transport, which are mitochondrial density and muscle's ability to oxidize fatty acids. If the mitochondrial is too dense, the fatty acids will encounter difficulty entering the organelles. Additionally, if a muscle is not properly conditioned to oxidize fatty acids, their use within the citric acid cycle is decreased. However, an increase in aerobic conditioning will improve fatty-acid oxidization.

Aerobic Conditioning Allows for Easier use of Fats as Fuel

Jeukendrip, Saris, and Wagenmakers (1998) went on to write Part II to their research on fat metabolism, "Fat Metabolism during Exercise: A review—Part II: Regulation of Metabolism and the Effects of Training." Part II examined lipolysis stimulation and suppression as well as exercise intensity's influence on fatty acids. The research uncovered that catecholamines, which are a basic compound acting as a hormone or neurotransmitter, stimulate lipolysis whereas insulin suppresses lipolysis. Jeukendrip, Saris, and Wagenmakers stated low- to moderate-intensity exercise is shown to increase lipolysis. Once exercise intensity increases, lipolysis occurs at a lower rate. Moreover, increasing intensity produces a reduction in fatty-acid availability as well as changes intramuscular factors that decrease fat oxidization. Additionally, fatty acid oxidization increases after exercise occurs intramuscularly due to an increase in oxidative enzymes and mitochondrial density.

A Higher Percentage of Fat is Used as Fuel During Lower Intensity Activity

After performing the first two reviews on fat metabolism, Jeukendrip, Saris, and Wagenmakers (1998) went on to write part III, "Fat Metabolism during Exercise: A Review—Part III: Effects of Nutritional Interventions." The purpose of this study is whether nutritional intervention can manipulate fat oxidation. They learned that by manipulating fat intake through supplementation, it is possible to increase fat oxidation; however, manipulating fat intake through supplementation is not suggested due to gastronomical distress. Furthermore, taking doses low enough to avoid gastronomical distress are minute and not worthwhile.

Jeukendrup (2002) continued his research on the regulation of fat metabolism in skeletal muscle and discovered skeletal muscle fat metabolism is multifactorial and involves an array of mechanisms varying on the conditions. Furthermore, increasing the rate at which molecules pass through the glycolytic pathway may decrease fat metabolism. This discovery plays into the mobilization and transport of fatty acids. If glycolysis is happening readily then fat metabolism is not as imperative.

High Intensity Exercise Relies Primarily on the Phosphagen and Glycolysis System

Research by Friedlander et al. (2007) on the contributions of working muscles to whole-body lipid metabolism found similar results to Jeukendrip and colleagues (1998) work. Over a nine-week period, Friedlander et al. studied eight male subjects to examine the effects of exercise intensity and endurance training five days per week, one hour per day at 75 percent VO₂peak exercise session. Friedlander and colleagues established most lipid oxidation occurs at low intensity, 62 percent lipid oxidation. Whereas 30 percent of lipid oxidation occurs during high-intensity exercise. What's more, free fatty-acid uptake and lipid oxidation increase from untrained to trained athletes.

Stallnect, Dela, and Helge (2007) carried out research on the topic of blood flow and lipolysis and found that although the process of "spot reduction" or burning fat in a specific region by target training that area may have some truth behind it after all. Although spot reduction is a myth, Stallnecht et al. discovered "spot lipolysis" in adipose tissue occurring when blood flow and lipolysis are higher in subcutaneous adipose tissue muscles adjacent to contracting muscles than in adjacent resting muscles, regardless of exercise intensity. The study involved ten healthy individuals performing one-legged knee extension exercises. After the exercises were performed, the participants' blood flow was estimated as well as their lipolysis calculated. Findings showed an increase in both blood flow and lipolysis in muscles adjacent to muscles that were contracting during the one-leg extension exercise more than in muscles adjacent to muscles that were not contracting.

Percentage of Fat Metabolism is Higher in Exercising than Non-Exercising Muscles

Readily available fatty acids for energy metabolism show their value through providing substrate for exercise. Therefore, lipid supplementation and its utilization during exercise in proportion to its content are worth investigation. Work by Zehnder et al. (2006) examines the effectiveness of providing more intramyocellular lipids during the last 1.5 days of a four-day diet on eleven endurance-trained males consuming a high-carbohydrate low-fat diet for the first 2.5 days of their diet. Since intramyocellular lipids and muscle glycogen provide local energy during exercise, Zehnder and colleagues wanted to know if the additional fat intake would increase intramyocellular lipids and thus improve performance. Results revealed the increase in fat intake during the last 1.5 days of the diet increased intramyocellular lipids that decrease in proportion to their initial content partly in exchange for peripheral fatty acids, which are used in the citric acid cycle.

A study by Knechtle, Baumann, Wirth, Knechtle, and Rosemann (2010) examined male ironman triathletes to determine if during an Ironman triathlon, they lose body mass in the form of fat mass or skeletal muscle mass. Upon gathering results from twenty-seven Caucasian, nonprofessional male Ironman triathletes, Knechtle and colleagues discovered males lose 1.8 kg of body mass and 1 kg of skeletal-muscle mass during an Ironman triathlon. These findings are thought to be due to a depletion of intramyocellular stored glycogen and lipids.

Research by Melanson, Gozansky, Barry, Maclean, Grunwald, and Hill (2009) investigated if when energy balance is maintained, exercise effects fat oxidation and fat balance in lean sedentary, lean endurance-trained, and obese sedentary men and women. Participants were asked to exercise for one hour on a stationary bike at 55 percent of aerobic capacity. Measurements were taken on twenty-four-hour glucose, insulin, and free fatty-acid profiles. Results were similar for exercise and nonexercise days. However, after consumption of the first meal, free fatty-acid concentrations remained below fasting levels for the remainder of the day. These findings suggest when exercise is performed with energy replacement, a.k.a energy balance, is maintained; twenty-four-hour fat oxidation does not increase and, in fact, may be slightly decreased.

Calorie Supplementation During Exercise Delays Our Use of Fat as Fuel

A study by Larson-Meyer, Redman, Heilbronn, Martin, and Ravussin (2010) looks to find an answer to the age-old debate over the independent effects of aerobic fitness and body fatness on morality and disease risk. Larson-Meyer et al. developed a study to determine if a 25 percent energy deficit yielded by calorie restriction or calorie restriction plus exercise will have the same effects on fat mass, visceral fat, VO₂peak, muscular strength, blood lipids, blood pressure, and insulin sensitivity/secretion. After six months results showed that VO₂peak was significantly improved in the calorie-restricted plus exercise group and not in the calorie-restricted group. Muscular strength did not change for either group. There were also no differences between losses of weight, fat mass, visceral fat, and systolic blood pressure amid the two groups. However, the calorie-restricted plus exercise group underwent a significant decrease in diastolic blood pressure, low-density lipoprotein cholesterol, and a significant increase in insulin sensitivity. These finding suggest that although calorie restriction alone leads to fat loss, aerobic fitness as well as improved insulin sensitivity, low-density lipoprotein cholesterol, and diastolic blood pressure all improved with the addition of exercise.

The following study by Redman, Heilbronn, Martin, Alfonso, Smith, Ravussin, Pennington, and CALERIE Team (2007) was conducted to examine the effects of calorie restriction with or without exercise on body composition and fat distribution. A randomized controlled trial consisting of thirty-six overweight but otherwise healthy participants (sixteen males and nineteen females) was established to test the effect of a 25 percent energy deficit by diet alone or diet plus exercise over a six-month period on body composition and fat distribution. Participants either a control group consisting of a healthy weight-maintenance diet, calorie restriction with a 25 percent reduction in energy intake, or calorie restriction plus exercise broken into a 12.5 percent reduction in energy intake plus a 12.5 percent increase in exercise energy expenditure. Findings showed no difference between the calorie-restricted group and calorie-restricted plus exercise group. Both groups lost roughly 10 percent of body weight, 24 percent of fat mass, and 27 percent of abdominal visceral fat suggesting calorie restriction is as good as calorie restriction plus exercise on body composition and fat distribution. Although exercise may produce additional fitness benefits that calorie restriction alone does not provide.

There Are Benefits to Exercise That Calorie Restriction Alone Does Not Provide

Goto, Ishii, Sugihara, Yoshioka, and Takamatsu (2007) set out to discover the effects of prior resistance exercise on lipolysis during subsequent submaximal exercise with different recovery periods between bouts. Participants were ten male subjects performing three types of exercise regimen. The first consisted of endurance exercise only. The second was submaximal endurance exercise with prior resistance exercise and twenty minutes of rest between resistance exercise and endurance exercise. The third exercise regimen was submaximal endurance exercise with prior resistance exercise and 120 minutes of rest between resistance exercise and endurance exercise. Submaximal endurance exercise was performed at 50 percent VO_2max on the cycle ergometer. The resistance exercise was six exercises with three to four sets of ten repetitions maximum. Results showed prior exercise caused increases in blood lactate, plasma norepinephrine, serum growth hormone, insulin, and glycerol concentrations. With that said, lipolysis was observed only in the trial with shorter rest (twenty minutes) between resistance exercise and submaximal exercise bouts.

Reduced Rest Between Sets Utilizes More Fat as Fuel

A study by Walts, Hanson, Delmonico, Yao, Wang, and Hurley (2008) looks to learn if sex or race differences influence strength training effects on muscle or fat specifically on thigh muscle volume, midthigh subcutaneous fat, and intermuscular fat. The study was composed of 181 previously inactive healthy participants (Caucasian, N = 117; African American, N = 54; Women, N = 99). Before and after ten weeks of strength training via unilateral knee extensions quadriceps muscle volume, midthigh subcutaneous fat, and intermuscular fat cross-sectional area were measured. Findings revealed training promotes greater increase in muscle volume in men than women, although percentages of muscle-volume increase were similar. There were no significant differences in muscle volume between races. There were no significant changes in subcutaneous fat or intermuscular fat. These results suggest sex or racial differences do not alter subcutaneous fat or intermuscular fat.

Further research by Zehnder, Ith, Kreis, Saris, Boutellier, and Boesch (2005) examined gender-specific differences in usage of intramyocellular lipids and glycogen utilization during exercise. Nine males and nine females had their intramyocellular lipids and glycogen as well as total fat and carbohydrate oxidation measured before, during, and after an endurance exercise consisting of up to three hours at 50 percent maximal workload for trained participants. Results showed average fat oxidation was the same for men and women, whereas carbohydrate oxidation was significantly higher in males compared to females. However, relative contribution of these substrates to total energy used were similar in males and females.

All Races and Genders Metabolize Substrates Relatively the Same

Overall, the above studies provide an array of findings concerning exercise physiology. Therefore, it is best to discuss the findings in two subgroups. First, nutrition. A few interesting findings arouse regarding nutrition's metabolic role in exercise. The primary takeaway being sustaining adequate amounts of nutrients in appropriate ratios with proper timing keeps the body performing at a higher rate for longer periods. With this said, glycolytic supplemental intervention is preferred over manipulating fat intake due to gastronomical distress. Moreover, by supplementing glucose an energy substrate switch can occur raising the rate of energy provide to working muscle to a higher ratio of glucose than fatty acids when fatty acids may otherwise have been utilized.

During Exercise, Glucose Supplementation is Recommended Over Fat Consumption

The second subgroup to discuss is exercise parameters ranging from type, intensity, duration, frequency, and rest. Exercise parameters affect mechanisms of the body on a global scale. For instance, increasing aerobic conditioning improves fatty acid oxidation. The intensity of exercise has a direct effect on lipolysis, lower-intensity exercise requiring a higher rate of lipolysis than high-intensity exercise. Endurance exercise such as during an ironman competition can result in a reduction in skeletal muscle mass during a single instance of the activity. Exercise causes immense alterations to the body. Types of exercise even affect each other's influence on the body if performed in close enough period.

Concurrently Using Two Training Modalities in a Single Session Alters Each Modalities

All in all, nutritional intervention and exercise parameters have a strong partnership when it comes to metabolic responses of the body. Research even showed calorie restriction and exercise leading to a calorie deficit to have similar outcomes on fat and weight loss. Not to mention, nutritional and exercise outcomes were shown to be independent of race or gender.

After examining the above literature, exercise is a dynamic process influenced by several seemingly independent yet highly correlated systems. Parameters of fitness such as type, intensity, duration, frequency, and rest all affect the endocrine system response to an equal degree as chemical reactions initiated through nutritional intervention. The body's response as an adaptive organic system to exercise, endocrinology, and nutritional intervention governs the adaptive form the body undertakes to best utilize its resources to better itself for future athletic endeavors.

Neuromuscular physiology examines the mechanisms affecting central nervous system (CNS) and peripheral nervous system (PNF) responses influencing perception and human motor behavior in humans. These influences are either acute (arousal, fatigue, and sleep) or chronic (aging, disease, training, and learning) (ufl.edu 2014). Human movement is a product of perception and behavior. Perception is how the body understands what is occurring, and behavior is its physiological response to its perception of the event. Perception spawns a behavior that, in turn, cultivates a new perception leading to yet another new behavior. This process is how human movement patterns are developed (Cook 2010, 269). These perceptions and behaviors are elicited by signals activated during movement. Some theorist believe these signals to be part of the central nervous system (brain and spinal cord) and others belief they occur because of mechanisms within the peripheral nervous system (extremities). Still others have an idea that a combination of CNS and PNS are responsible for regulating human movement.

The next two chapters search through a variety of research concerning the controlling mechanisms of skeletal-muscle fatigue to determine if science has concluded as to whether CNS, PNS, or both is responsible for exercise induced fatigue within the neuromuscular system. The frontier of human athletic potential resides in understanding the mechanisms restraining athletes from achieving absolute athleticism. Although there are numerous elements responsible for athletic progress, the most substantial mechanism impeding athletes from reaching ever-higher levels of athletic ability is fatigue.

Legendary coach Vince Lombardi once said, "fatigue makes cowards of us all." Regardless of the fitness component being stressed (muscular and cardiovascular endurance, strength, or power), fatigue is always the limiting factor. Athletes invest countless hours physically training to push back the point at which fatigue stops them from further activity. Fatigue renders athletes motionless and unable to perform their task any longer. Avoiding fatigue is the goal of every athlete. Physical activity and exercise was traditionally believed to be limited by a peripherally based, metabolite-induced failure of the contractile function of skeletal muscle, independent of muscle inhibition by the central nervous system (CNS). Fatigue induced within skeletal muscle is known as peripheral fatigue. The theory of peripheral fatigue as the cause of fatigue during exercise is known as catastrophe theory (Noakes 2007).

Catastrophe Theory Implies Fatigue is Induced Within Muscles

Over decades, catastrophe theory has evolved as technology has improved scientific research. Beginning in the 1920s, decades prior to what catastrophe theory is today, Sir Archibald Vivian Hill and his colleagues proposed performance during exercise of high intensity was limited by skeletal-muscle anaerobiosis due to limited skeletal-muscle blood flow, following myocardial ischemia. Hill believed the skeletal-muscle anaerobiosis prevented the neutralization of the lactic acid that initiated muscle contraction. The accumulation of lactic acid impaired skeletal-muscle relaxation and eventually caused muscle failure and eventual cessation of activity. Hill's model eventually evolved into Richard Edwards's catastrophe theory that is the leading model of fatigue. Edwards's modern catastrophe theory is based on the notion that human movement ceases when there is a catastrophic failure of homoeostasis in the local musculature (Noakes and St. Clair Gibson 2004). When skeletal muscle contraction terminates, it is local to the muscle worked and its ability to supply energy substrate or clear acidosis metabolite.

A revolutionary theory challenges conventional thought and catastrophe theory, designating the central nervous system as the limiting factor ensuring overphysical exertion does not lead to catastrophic physiological failure during physical activity (Noakes, St. Clair Gibson, Lambert 2004). This new model is known as the central governor model (CGM). Central governor model was first introduced by Timothy D. Noakes and colleagues.

According to Central governor model, exercise is limited by "central" fatigue from feed-forward mechanisms and afferent feedback from varying physiological systems. The central nervous system uses afferent information from the peripheral nervous system to halt exercise before catastrophe strikes preventing damaging effects to the body (Noakes 2007; Lambert, St. Clair Gibson, Noakes 2005). Under the theory of central governor model, exercise is stopped prior to the occurrence of absolute catastrophe. This central nervous system fatigue regulator is believed to be an ancient genetic safety mechanism put in place and passed down through generations keeping people safe from working so intensely that they would tear tendons from bone, explode their heart, or burst a lung (Hopkins 2009). Although the central governor model's purpose is to keep the body from destroying itself, athletic progress is founded in pushing back fatigue and driving progress. Therefore, sports and exercise science must identify safe methods of hacking the central governor model to prolong physical activity.

The following critical review examines Timothy Noakes's central governor model and Mihaly Csikszentmihalyi's flow as a psychological instrument in overriding the central governor and pushing back fatigue by being so immersed in the activity that the central nervous system is not using its afferent feedback to stop physical activity (Csikszentmihalyi 1990; Kayser 2003). The review will begin with a brief overview of the central governor model including supporting and opposing stands on central governor model's validity (Noakes and Marino 2009; Shepard 2009). Following the central governor model review, research concerning flow's place in exercise and sports will be examined with the purpose of immersing athletes in flow longer and more often to push back fatigue and increase performance. Then an examination of flow in areas outside of exercise and sport will be reviewed to derive crossover findings from non-exercise-related research findings to extract flow instigating methods for exercise and sport.

Central governor model validity

The first study examines the central nervous system's role in skeletal muscle fatigue asking the question directly: is fatigue all in your head? Weir, Beck, Cramer, and Housh (2006) review a body of knowledge concerning the central governor model. They suggest that the subconscious brain regulates power output (pacing strategy) by modulating motor-unit recruitment to preserve whole-body homeostasis and prevent catastrophic physiological failure. The central governor model defines fatigue as a sensation or emotion as opposed to a decline in the ability to produce force or power. The argument supporting the central governor model is that lactic acid models do not accurately account for fatigue; therefore, something beyond peripheral-based fatigue models must be presiding over fatigue. A central nervous system-based pacing strategy would account for fatigue where lactic acid models fall apart. I will cover lactic acid in the next chapter.

Evidence of central governor model is made present in a study by Swart, Lamberts, Lambert,Clair Gibson, Lambert, Skowno, and Noakes (2009). The study was established to determine if there is a protective mechanism put in place by the central nervous system to regulate prolonged exercise performance protecting athletes from pushing themselves so far;

they leave homeostasis and enter a state of emergency. Participants were eight elite cyclists instructed to ingest ten milligrams of methylphenidate (a stimulant) in a randomized placebo-controlled crossover trail and a placebo group that did not ingest the methylphenidate. After ingesting the methylphenidate, participants were instructed to cycle for a given period until their power output fell to 70 percent of their starting value. The results showed the group receiving methylphenidate cycled for approximately 32 percent longer than the placebo group. Swart and colleagues concluded that because the cyclists were able to push beyond their natural boundaries with the aid of a stimulant, there is a reserve in place for maintaining whole-body homeostasis in case of emergency. These findings suggest that because there is always a reserve present allowing athletes to push beyond a peripheral nervous system-based upper limit, the central nervous system is the true governor of fatigue. Accepting afferent feedback from the peripheral nervous system to determine when to initiate fatigue.

Central Governor Model Suggest Fatigue Keeps Us from Harming Ourselves

Another study supporting the central governor model as fatigue's determinant was completed by Hargreaves (2008) and looks toward glucose interaction with the central nervous system and its effect on fatigue. The greatest finding of Hargreaves research is that the simple presence of carbohydrates in the oral cavity may interact with the central nervous system to prolong performance. Hargreaves brings a quote from a 1925 Boston marathon runner to attention, "Every time I ate a piece of candy I felt fresh." The marathon runner's statement points out that the presence of glucose in an athlete's mouth triggers that individual to take more from his or her energy reserve with the expectation that more glucose is coming shortly (an individual piece of candy does not supply enough glucose to have a significant effect on energy substrate during a marathon). This is hinting that the central nervous system is regulating glucose use in the peripheral nervous system though feed-forward mechanisms and afferent feedback. To further illustrate Hargreaves findings, Hargreaves focuses on a quote by Finnish runner Paavo Nurmi, "Mind is everything, muscles pieces of rubber. All that I am. I am because of my mind." In other words, Paavo Nurmi is saying, the limits of the body are put in place by the mind. If the simple presence of glucose in an athlete's mouth can prolong exercise without adding any substantial amount of glucose to the muscles, that is substantial evidence that the central nervous system is regulating muscle's work capacity.

CNS Theories of Fatigue State the Limits of the Body Are Set by the Mind

Additional fatigue models

There are three other additional fatigue models worth bringing to attention. Research by Weir, Beck, Cramer, and Housh (2006) suggest the central governor model does not fully explain fatigue. Just as the peripheral-based models of fatigue have its flaws, the central governor model also has unanswered questions. Weir and his colleagues suggest task dependency model is a more encompassing model of fatigue. Suggesting the central nervous system and peripheral nervous system work synergistically to monitor fatigue during varying task. Task dependency model's strength relies on the thought that the body functions as a synergistic mechanism, not the combination of independent isolated activities.

Task Dependency Model States the CNS and PNS Work Synergistically

Research by Barry and Enoka (2007) states that perhaps a task-failure model is responsible for fatigue. Barry and Enoka's task-failure approach involves comparing two performances and identifying the adjustments that limit the rate for the more difficult condition. According to task-failure approach, a sustained contraction can be influenced by such variables as the type of load supported by the limb, the posture of the limb, and the group of muscles involved in the task. However, task-failure approach has challenges as well. The main challenge being identifying the mechanisms enabling these different variables to influence the time-to-task failure.

Task-Failure Model Suggest the Exercise Modality is Responsible for Fatigue

Another model of brain regulation of physical performance is the psychobiological model. The psychobiological model states that if the perception of fatigue outweighs motivation, you will slow down or stop. According to this model, it is our relationship between sensation of fatigue and our motivation that makes the difference (Marcora 2008).

Psychobiological Model States Motivation Keeps Fatigue at Bay

Flow's role

With sufficient evidence supporting the central nervous system's role in controlling fatigue and performance, an examination of flow's role in improving athletic performance through central nervous system manipulation can be examined. Flow is a well-known phenomenon in sports, flow most commonly referred to by athletes as "being in the zone" (Csikszentmihalyi, 2012). Flow tends to occur when a person faces a clear set of goals requiring appropriate responses such as what is found in sports. It is easy to enter flow in sports because they have goals and rules making it possible for the player to act without questioning what and how a task should be done. For the duration of the sporting event, the player lives in a self-contained universe unaware of his or her outside surroundings or even internal emotions such as happiness. Achieving flow is key to reaching athletic potential. With that said, the study of flow is of great importance to athletes. The following research examines flow during athletic environments to learn what brings about enhanced flow states while exercising and training for sports and how these flow states can be enhanced. As well as factors that diminish the chances of an athlete entering flow.

Jackson (1992) conducted a qualitative investigation in the flow experiences of elite figure skaters. Jackson performed the study to gain greater insight into the nature of flow in sport. Participants were sixteen former US national-champion figure skaters, holding their titles between 1985 and 1990. The participants were interviewed on an optimal skating experience and then questioned extensively regarding factors associated with achieving optimal or flow states during performance. Factors perceived as most important for getting into flow included a positive mental attitude, positive precompetitive and competitive affect, maintaining appropriate focus, physical readiness, and, for some pairs dance skaters, unity with their partner. Factors that were perceived to disrupt or prevent flow include physical problems/mistakes, an inability to maintain focus, a negative mental attitude, and lack of audience response. Jackson found the skater's description of what was occurring during optimal skating were similar to characteristics of flow. The skaters were in a positive state during flow, and negative mental-states disrupted their flow. This makes sense, since people generally associate flow with the ability to perform task that otherwise would be difficult or impossible.

To Engage in Flow, Skill and Challenge Must be in Harmony

These findings illustrate that drawing on experience of elite athletes may improve understanding of flow in sports. If researchers can discover what elite athletes are experiencing as they enter and experience flow, they may be able to develop methods for nonelite athletes to increase their flow experience while exercising for pleasure, training for competition, and during competition.

Additional research of flow in sports looks at three potential psychological antecedents of flow in sports: goals, competence, and confidence. Stein, Kimiecik, Daniels, and Jackson (1995) examine tennis players competing in weekend tournaments, basketball players in college activity classes, and golf regulars. Participants of the first group rated flow characteristics, whereas the second and third groups used the experience sampling method to measure flow. Stein and colleagues discovered that in learning environments (basketball classes), students in flow experienced greater enjoyment satisfaction, concentration, and control than their counterparts experiencing boredom, apathy, or anxiety. Students in the competitive environments (tennis tournament and golf) noted that while in flow or boredom states, they had a better quality of experience than individuals in apathy or anxiety states.

These findings suggest contextual differences influence why an athlete perceives a situation as optimal. The psychological antecedents of flow for sport participants remain unidentified, as neither goals, competence, nor confidence predicted the flow experience. However, valuable information was unearth regarding context of the situation. Athletes, coaches, and sporting administers can take these findings and use their gained knowledge making alterations to the context of the sporting event improving an athlete's experience.

A study by Kowal and Fortier (2010) examined the relationships between different types of situational motivation and flow and situational motivational determinants (perceptions of autonomy, competence, and relatedness) and the experience of flow. Participants were 203 master-level swimmers who immediately following a swim practice completed a questionnaire assessing different variables. Results showed that situational, self-determined forms of motivation (intrinsic motivation and self-determined, extrinsic motivation) and perceptions of autonomy, competence, and relatedness were positively related to flow, whereas amotivation was negatively related to flow. These findings suggest athletes will enter a deeper and longer state of flow when participating in sports of their choosing because of intrinsic motivators they feel are important as opposed to extrinsic motivators their coach, teammates, or parents may be pressuring them toward. In other words, an athlete's desire to participate in sport is a significant factor in their success.

Success Follows Desire and Desire Stems from Past Success

Flow in non-sport activities

There is a great wealth of research on flow in domains outside of exercise and sport that can aid athletes in attaining a state of flow. The following portion of this chapter will examine what initiates flow in numerous activities outside of sports and what we can take away from these insights to improve ease into flow, frequency, duration, and intensity during exercise.

The pioneer of flow Mihaly Csikszentmihalyi has unearth countless determinants of flow, one important aspect being creativity. Csikszentmihalyi (2013) explores creativities embodiment in flow. Creativity according to Csikszentmihalyi takes rise from the interaction of three elements: a culture containing symbolic rules, a person bringing novelty into the symbolic domain, and a field of experts recognizing and validating the innovation. These three elements are also evident in sports domains. With respect to sports, the elements can be broken down into a governing body overseeing the sports organization and setting rules and culture to the organization, the athlete who brings novel actions into the sporting domain, and a field of experts ranging from referees, umpires, judges, and fans who recognize and validate the innovation. By looking at sports in this manner, sports are clearly a domain for cultivating creativity and, in turn, nurturing flow.

Sports are a Perfect Domain for Sparking Creativity

Moreover, people naturally possess two distinct traits. "A conservative tendency, made up of instincts for self-preservation, self-aggrandizement, and saving energy, and an expansive tendency made up of instincts for exploring, for enjoying novelty and risk" (Csikszentmihalyi 2013). The second traits consisting of instincts for exploring and for enjoying novelty and risk are traits common among athletes. Athlete's by nature are pushing boundaries, taking risk, and exploring novel methods of training and competing. The very nature of an athlete's purpose embellishes her sport through the creative process taking place during the basic act of sport participation.

Athletes as a Demographic Enjoy Exploring, Novelty, and Risk

With this said, the elements of creativity influencing flow are also evident in sports. Creativity allows athletes to immerse themselves in the activity and act without thinking or by instinct, which is a key characteristic of flow (Kotler 2014). By inspiring creativity, flow is encouraged and is the heart of athletic success. Creativity is seen during every amazing play, match, or other accomplishment during sports. The athletes could lose themselves in the moment and let their knowledge and experience carry them to success. Athletes are creative masterminds in their own sense, reaching a state of flow allows that creativity to flourish.

One of the most important yet difficult places to attain flow is the classroom. That is why Shernoff et al. (2003) investigated a 526-participant sample of student engagement based upon flow traits (concentration, interest, and enjoyment). Shernoff and colleagues examined how adolescents spent their time in high school and the conditions under which they reported being engaged. Participants experienced increased engagement when they perceived challenge of the task and their own skills were high and in balance, the instruction was relevant, and the learning environment was under their control. Results also revealed participants were also more engaged in individual and group work versus listening to lectures, watching videos, or taking exams.

Active Participation is More Productive than Passive Involvement

These findings suggest increasing engagement by focusing on learning activities that provide an appropriate level of challenge for student skills. Taking this data and interpreting it for athletes, we have learned that during times that are traditionally considered difficult to attain participant engagement such as a classroom setting, by ensuring skills match the challenge and a sense of autonomy are present, engagement is more likely to occur. Exercise settings can take this knowledge and apply it by establishing an environment where participants are challenged at a level appropriate for their skill. Exercise participants should also voice their opinion regarding components of exercise such as primary focus of exercise activity, exercise selection, and intensity if they are to fully engage themselves in the activity.

Online games and flow in classrooms

On the opposing end of the spectrum from classrooms, online games have proven to be a highly profitable e-commerce application for years. Bringing in large numbers of online players. Hsu and Lu (2003) know the reasons why people volunteer and enjoy playing online games is an important area of research. Hsu and Lu apply the technology acceptance model (TAM) that incorporates social influences and flow experience as belief-related constructs to predict users' acceptance of online games. The technology acceptance model was empirically evaluated using survey data collected from 233 users about their perceptions of online games. Results of the survey showed that social norms, attitude, and flow experience explain about 80 percent of game playing. Comparing the findings of Hsu and Lu to those of Shernoff and colleagues flow appears to be almost a given in online games whereas engagement (a flow state) is a yearning characteristic in classrooms having difficulty enticing students.

Classrooms can Learn from Videogames

These findings imply that characteristics of online games encourage a state of flow that classrooms do not. Chiang, Lin, Cheng, and Liu (2011) believe online gaming has many features encouraging flow states, including the provision of rich and immediate feedback to player actions, enjoyment, playfulness, and the ability to induce high levels of player concentration. Moreover, a study by Stein, Kimiecik, Daniels, and Jackson (1995) found flow experience occurs more often when participants freely choose to enter an activity such as online games whereas school is mandatory and more challenging to enter flow state. I have also published peer-reviewed research on gamification's ability to increase attraction, participation, and retention in adventure and wilderness sports, and I found game-based mechanics to be a valuable tool in motivating athletes. These positive flow states should be promoted to establish a culture rich in the flow cultivating characteristics apparent in online games.

Game-Based Mechanics Improve Attraction, Participation, and Retention in Sports

Food's role

Another study focusing on CNS's nutritional considerations is "Serotonin and Central Nervous System Fatigue: Nutritional Considerations" (2000). It has been known that the neurotransmitter serotonin (5-hydroxytryptamine (5-HT) has been linked to increased physical and perhaps mental fatigue during endurance exercise. Davis, Alderson, and Welsh (2000) are investigating whether ingestion of carbohydrates (CHO) and branched-chain amino acids (BCAA) will alter the metabolism of brain 5-HT by affecting the availability of its amino-acid precursor. Thus, lowering the availability of 5-HT in the brain and delaying physical and mental fatigue. What Davis et al. discovered is that although CHO ingestion does delay physical and mental fatigue, BCAA were not shown to delay physical and mental fatigue. The authors concluded that for BCAAs to be effective in reducing fatigue, large doses that can slow water absorption across the gut, cause gastrointestinal disturbances, and decrease fluid palatability are required. Davis and his colleagues further noted that now it is difficult to tell if the increase ingestion of CHO is delaying fatigue due to its role in the CNS or its availability in the PNS. Further research into this topic may yield a clearer answer. Davis's research is a step forward in nutrition, brain neurochemistry, and fatigue's role in sports-and-exercise performance enhancement. By having a better understanding of nutrition's role in athletic performance, athletes have increased opportunity to enhanced training and performance outcomes.

Carbohydrates Keep Fatigue at Bay Better Than BCAAs

Overall

Thus, the central governor model whether the sole predict of athletic ability or part of an intrinsic system synergistically working together with the peripheral system to keep the body in homeostasis when pushed to its limits is a model worth further investigation. With that said, flow's impact on the central governor model, specifically an individual's engagement in an activity and resilience to fatigue during exercise, appears to be an advantageous method for athletes to engage their minds so deeply in the athletic endeavor at hand that the barrier of fatigue is pushed back, regardless if it is physiological, psychological, or psycholobiological. By discovering methods of engrossing athletes deeply in their activity to the extent that conscious and unconscious acknowledgment of fatigue is overridden, the limits of athletic potential can be lifted. If we can improve methods of increasing flow's ease of entry, frequency, intensity, and duration by utilizing traits that athletes encounter during immense physical activity that emerges them in flow and that nonathletes encounter during activities that bring them into a flow state, then the limits of fatigue can be diminished, and the boundaries of athletic achievement can be raised to unprecedented levels. There are numerous theories regarding the mind as the limiting factor in physical fatigue and performance decline. Regardless of which models are true, if one of them is correct it would mean your potential as an athlete is highly influenced by your will to succeed. With that said, let's examine the traditional model of fatigue.

Shifting gears from the CNS's role over fatigue is the more traditional stance of peripheral system's function as the determining factor governing fatigue. Research examining PNSs part with fatigue examines the biochemistry of exercise-induced metabolic acidosis. The investigation coordinated by Robergs, Ghiasvand, and Parker (2004) is an overview of research going against the historical notion of lactate production causing acidosis. As scientific instruments improve with technology, scientists reveal more accurate portrayals of how the human body functions. Roberg's study showcases ATP breakdown into ADP and P(i) as the new model of acidosis within a muscle. Every time ATP is broken down into ADP and P(i), a proton is released. It is this proton release causing acidosis and fatigue. If the demand of muscle contraction is met by mitochondrial respiration, proton presence is at homeostasis within the muscle. As more ATP is needed to form new energy during glycolysis and the phosphagen system, more protons are released, thus a greater burning sensation and fatigue. While the protons are being released during glycolysis, lactate is being produced at the same time to prevent pyruvate accumulation and supply the NAD(+) needed for phase two of glycolysis. Therefore, although lactate production is not a direct cause of acidosis, it occurs at the same time and is a proper marker. Sports scientist can use this knowledge to indirectly track fatigue resistance in athletes by tracking lactate.

An in-depth examination of the production of lactate in human skeletal muscles during exercise from an enzymatic approach was undergone by Spriet, Howlett, and Heigenhauser (2000). The purpose of their research was to investigate the production of lactate in human skeletal muscle over a range of power outputs. Lactate production is dictated by pyruvate and NADH levels, which are in turn related to exercise intensity. Higher-exercise intensity brings about increased levels of pyruvate and NADH. What Spriet, Howlett, and Heigenhauser results found is lactate production is positively correlated with exercise intensity. Lower power outputs yielded little or no lactate production.

Lactate's role as an energy source make its presence in muscles desired. Furthermore, Brooks (2000) gave the "lactate shuttle hypothesis," which states lactate plays a key role in the distribution of carbohydrates potential energy that occurs among various tissue and intra- and extracellular compartments. Further hammering the importance of lactate as a useful metabolite through the body and not a hindering by-product.

Lactate Distributes Energy Throughout the Body

Additional research performed by Gladden (2000) highlighted muscle's role as a consumer of lactate. It has been known for some time that muscles are a producer of lactate, but Gladden's research shows muscles consume lactate according to metabolic rate, blood flow, lactate concentration, hydrogen ion concentration, fiber type, and exercise training. Gladden presumed muscles most likely consume more lactate during steady-state exercise because of increased lactate oxidation. The research also noted that oxidative muscle fibers are metabolically suited for lactate transport more so than glycolytic muscle fibers. Furthermore, endurance-trained muscles oxidize lactate better and have a better capacity for sarcolemmal lactate transport.

Lactate Clears More Easily During Aerobic Activity

Building upon the consumption of lactate in muscles, Donovan and Pagliassotti (2000) took lactate disposal a step further and quantitatively assessed the pathways for lactate disposal in skeletal-muscle fiber types. Donovan and Pagliassotti's findings suggest fiber type does indeed influence the pathways for lactate disposal. Type I and type IIa muscle fibers use oxidization as the primary route of disposal, accounting for approximately 50 percent of the lactate removal. Type IIb muscle fiber's primary pathway for lactate disposal was gluconeogenesis. Donovan and Pagliassotti also discovered that gluconeogenesis capacity was the same for type IIa and type IIb fiber types. What this means for practical application is using active recovery, which is primarily an oxidative activity used between high intensity sets during exercise, is a good means to dispose of lactate when it needs to be reduced within a muscle, and the type II muscle fibers are limited by gluconeogenesis capacity.

Active Recovery Between Exercise Bouts Accelerates Lactate Clearance

If you're an athlete, chances are you have heard of the terms "lactic threshold" and "anaerobic threshold" (now more commonly referred to as "ventilation threshold" because you are not truly absent of oxygen but rather producing a greater amount of CO_2 relative to O_2 and exhalation becomes more forceful, thus eventually leading to exercise cessation). These two terms are often used interchangeably because they occur at almost the same time (lactic threshold occurring slightly before the ventilatory threshold). They are the result of two different yet related mechanisms.

The lactic threshold occurs slightly before the ventilatory threshold. When an athlete crosses over the lactic threshold, they are accumulating lactate in the muscles faster than the body can expel it back into the bloodstream.

Despite popular belief, lactic acid is not what causes the burning sensation in your muscles. The feeling is produced by a metabolite known as pyruvate. Pyruvate supplies energy while in an aerobic state, and once we cross over the ventilatory threshold, it undergoes fermentation resulting in lactate. Pyruvate's fermentation process is the product that leads to fatigue and that burning sensation.

Pyruvate Causes the Burning Sensation in Muscles

To manage pyruvate, your body begins a process of buffering that produces carbon dioxide and water as its by-products. The body must use ventilation to get rid of the high levels of carbon dioxide. It is at this point that we are trying so hard to get the carbon dioxide out that we cannot keep up with the amount of oxygen we need to bring in, hence excessive heavy breathing and further fatigue. See the diagram on the next page.

Crossing the Lactic Threshold

1

Aerobic = Pyruvate

2

Go Anaerobic > Fermentation Occurs > Produces Lactate > Acidosis & Metabolites > Cause Fatigue & Discomfort

Crossing the Ventilitory Threshold

3

Body Attempts to Buffer Pyruvate

=

Buffering Produces CO_2 & Water

4

Exhale Harder to Rid the Body of CO_2 > Cross Over Ventilitory Threshold > Causes Heavier Breathing > Enventual Slow Down or Bonk Because You Cannot Get in Enough O_2

As you can see, the harder you work, the more lactate, pyruvate, and carbon dioxide your body will produce, which will eventually lead to you stopping. Knowing this, training at or slightly below the ventilatory threshold and becoming better at removing lactate from the working muscles and thus raising the threshold, allowing for you to train at a higher level than you could maintain previously, is essential for endurance sports or sports involving repetitive bouts of sprinting.

Ventilatory Threshold Training Improves Repetitive Sprint Ability

The ventilation threshold is 80–90 percent of your MHR, which can easily be found via a heart rate monitor or by a simple talk test. With that said, heart rate monitors are prone to error and the chest straps are more accurate than wrist heart-rate monitors. If you don't have a chest strap heart-rate monitor and want to ensure accuracy, perform the talk test. If you can hold a conversation while exercising, you are below the threshold, and if you must take breaks to breathe, you have crossed the threshold.

A Simple Talk Test Can Let You Know You Are Performing Anaerobically

Moreover, "Skeletal Muscle Fatigue: Cellular Mechanisms" (2008) challenges the historical explanation of skeletal muscle fatigue. Under the notion, accumulation of intracellular lactate and hydrogen ions causing impaired function of the contractile proteins is most likely not the case for mammals. Allen and colleagues examine other possible explanations for fatigue such as the ionic changes on the action potential, failure of SR $Ca2+$ release by various mechanisms, and the effects of reactive oxygen species. Allen and colleagues make note that there are numerous contributing factors leading to fatigue, and it is important to identify the different mechanisms that contribute to fatigue under different circumstances.

Numerous Mechanisms Cause Fatigue

Another study up for review asks the question directly, is lactate production related to muscular fatigue? Macedo, Lazarim, Catanho, Tessuti, and Hohl (2009) conducted a study examining the cause-effect relationship between lactic acid, acidosis, and muscular fatigue. An experiment was devised by first-year university students consisting of two protocols of eight thirty-meter sprints at maximum speed. One protocol utilized 120-second rest intervals while the other protocol used 20-second rest intervals. The researchers were planning on using the experiment to answer three questions: (1) Which metabolic pathways of energy metabolism are responsible for meeting the high ATP demand during high-intensity intermittent exercise? (2) Which metabolic pathways are active during the pause, and how do they influence phosphocreatine synthesis? and (3) Is lactate production related to muscular fatigue? Once the experiment was complete, the participant's performance was analyzed. The students concluded that phosphocreatine restoration is time dependent, explaining the steady level of performance in the protocol consisting of 120-second rest intervals, whereas the 20-second rest interval protocol underwent performance detriment. The students also concluded that lactate production is not related to the performance decrement because the blood-lactate levels showed similar absolute increases after both performance decrements. Conveying these results to application in fitness, Macedo and his colleagues proved that although phosphocreatine restoration is time dependent and responsible for performance during intermittent thirty-meter sprints, blood-lactate levels are not. With that said, sport and fitness training protocols should use proper work to rest ratios when developing training protocols. The next page list common work-to-rest intervals for both rep and time-based training:

Rest Intervals Determine the Outcome of a Session as Much as Reps, Sets, and Weights

Work to Rest Intervals for Rep-Based Training

Repetitions	Rest
1-3	4-5 min
4-6	2-4 min
7-8	1 min
9-10	45-60 s
11-12	30-45 s
13-15+	< 30 s

Work to Rest Ratios for Time-Based Training

Activity	Ratio	Rest
5-10 s	1:6-1:12	1 min
15-30 s	1:3-1:4	1-1.5 min
1-3 min	1:1	1-3 min
3-5 min	1:1-2:1	1.5-5 min

*These are standard ratios. They can by altered if the workout has a "nonstandard" purpose.

The next two reviews dwell into PNS fatigue specific to local musculature biomechanics. The first one is "The Effects of Joint Angle on Electromyographic Indices of Fatigue" (2009), which was designed to examine the effect of manipulation on joint angle on electromyographic (EMG) fatigue curves at different sites of the quadriceps muscle group. The study consists of eight subjects performing isometric knee extensions at 0.26, 0.79, and 1.31 rad from full extension for one minute at 50 percent maximum effort. Electrode leads where placed over the vastus lateralis and vastus medialis to record EMG signals. The recordings were analyzed for changes in integrated EMG (IEMG), which were used to measure fatigue and median power frequency (MPF) over time. The findings suggest EMG responses where consistent over all sites, suggesting no variation in fatigue related to joint angle.

The Onset of Fatigue is Not Dependent on Joint Angle

The second of the two biomechanics focused studies of fatigue, "Effect of Fatigue on Hamstring Coactivation during Isokinetic Knee Extensions" (1998), examines the effect of fatigue of the quadriceps muscle on coactivation of the hamstring muscles and determined if the response is different between two isokinetic (constant) speeds. Coactivation occurs when the agonist and antagonist activate at the same time. Ten males and ten females with no known history of knee pathology performed fifty maximal knee extensions at two isokinetic speeds of 1.75 rad × s(−1) (100 degrees × s[−1]) and 4.36 rad × s(−1) (250 degrees × s([−1]). By interpreting electromyographic data recorded from the vastus lateralis and biceps femoris, more coactivation was apparent at higher speed; however, the increase in coactivation of the hamstring muscles was similar at both speeds.

The results of the above study deliver two intriguing findings. First, coactivation is greater at a higher isokinetic speed, and, second, coactivation increases during fatigue, but the rate of increase is independent of contraction velocity. What these discoveries mean for sports and exercise science is the common fitness model of training opposing muscle groups in a superset (two exercises performed back-to-back) fashion may not yield as adequate of a rest interval as once thought. With that said, personal trainers, physical therapist, and coaches should note the speed of muscle contraction during a given exercise when selecting a proper rest interval.

Increasing the Contraction Speed of a Muscle Induces Fatigue Sooner

Looking back, the above neuromuscular physiology reviews make it clear that there is no singular controlling mechanism responsible for skeletal muscle fatigue during exercise. Despite whether CNS or PNS is responsible for placing an upper limit on muscle contraction, there are numerous mechanisms involved throughout the process. Regardless if muscle contraction restriction is a technique devised by the brain to warn and stop athletic performance before damaging ramifications take place. Or if fatigue is a consequence of endangering homeostasis by provoking an acidosis condition within local musculature via over exertion. Fatigue occurs to keep the body safe before over exertion causes lasting damaging effects. For this reason, fatigue is worth a deeper examination into its mechanisms and process, especially flow's role in fatigue.

The better understanding personal trainers, physical therapist, and sports coaches are of fatigue's part in physical training and athletic competition, the safer they can train their athletes while yielding greater performance gains. When it comes to engineering athletes, safety is always priority. If athletes can safely enhance their performance, then athletic progress is able to leap to a new league. Comprehension of skeletal-muscle fatigue opens gateways to the next level of safely developing stronger, faster, and longer-lasting athletes.

One of the most common phrases I hear as a running coach and strength and conditioning coach is "I only want to work in my fat-burning zone because that burns the highest amount of fat." It's true that working in the fat-burning zone burns the highest percentage of calories from fat. However, it does not burn the most calories overall. With that said, I am going to clear up what each exercise zone does to your body, how to know when you are in each zone, and the benefits they provide.

Like any other element of fitness, runner's pace is influenced by numerous factors. Below are the main factors influencing a runner's pace:

Muscle Fiber Type: Not everyone is born to be an elite distance runner. There are two major fiber types: slow twitch (type I) and fast twitch (type II). Everyone has a combination of both fiber types, but people who are primarily slow twitch dominant are better at running slower longer distances, and people with a higher percentage of fast twitch are better at running faster shorter distances. Characteristics of each muscle type can be altered by doing the corresponding training. Muscle fibers can also increase in size by giving them the proper stress stimulus, heavy with long rest to increase the contractile filaments, and moderate with short rest to increase the metabolic component (read "How Muscle Is Made"). However, whether fiber types can be transformed is still a matter of debate.

Running Economy: Running economy is directly related to a runner's weight and gait and is a primary indicator of running performance. The less weight runners carry, the more energy they can save, thus use for running farther and faster. A runner's gait also affects running economy. The more efficient a runner's form, the more direct his movements will be and the better his running economy. Even if you are self-coached, it is a good idea to have your gait analyzed by a biomechanics expert who specializes in runners.

Fuel Utilization: During high-intensity aerobic activity (>70 percent VO$_2$max), the majority of energy comes from carbohydrates. However, through training this can be switched toward a higher fat-utilizing ratio. Fat has more energy than carbohydrates; therefore, the switch allows athletes to run further and faster since there is more energy available. Four hundred and sixty molecules of ATP (energy) are produced for every molecule of fat, whereas only thirty-six molecules of ATP are made for every molecule of carbohydrate. This means fat is twelve times more efficient than carbohydrates. The switch to better fat utilization can be triggered by running longer distances and performing ventilatory threshold training or exercising on a low-carb diet. Although medical clearance should be sought prior to any sever dietary restrictions during exercise. It is because fat is so much more efficient than carbohydrates that athletes need to take time training in a slow steady state prior to engaging in HIIT.

Fat is 12 Times More Efficient Than Carbohydrates

Each Training zone is reflected by a target heart rate range and associated benefits. The following is a chart listing training zones with corresponding purposes and outcomes of training in that zone.

Training Zones by Percent Max Heart Rate

Aerobic	Training Zone	Heart Rate Range (%)
	Warm-up	50-60
	Recovery Pace	60-70
	Base Building	70-80
Anaerobic	Race Pace	80-90
	VO$_2$max	92-98
	Repetition Pace	95-100

Warm-up: This zone is used for exactly what it's called, warming-up. It is performed between 50–60 percent of your max heart rate (MHR, fastest your heart can beat) and should be systemic (whole body). The more systemic the routine is, the shorter your warm-up can be. Remember, a warm-up for some could be a complete workout for others. Make sure you keep your heart rate in the correct region. Toward the end of the warm-up, heart rate should gradually build its way up to the focus training zone of the training session.

Recovery Pace: When we work in this zone, we are working at 60–70 percent of our MHR. This zone is popular because it is known as the fat-burning zone. However, while it is burning a higher percentage of fat, it is doing so at a significantly slower rate, this means you burn fewer calories overall and lose less weight in the end. While exercising in the fat-burning zone, you are primarily burning fat as energy, but because you are working more efficiently, consuming less oxygen, and activating less muscle, the total energy you are using is less. As you increase your effort, a higher percentage of energy comes from carbohydrates rather than fat, but you are burning more calories overall because calories are energy, and you need more energy to work at the higher intensity. The fat-burning zone can be more properly used for your recovery pace during metabolic workouts. When performing intervals, drop down to this pace for your recovery phase before raising it up again, or for the day before an exceptionally hard work out or race.

Base Building: The most fundamental aspect of metabolic training is building your base, yet far too often I see people struggling through intervals without a proper base built up first to help them sustain the high intensity of interval training. Yes, it is true; intervals are how you get faster. However, trying to perform quality intervals without a base is going to get you nowhere fast, please refer to the *PROformance Training Systems PROgression Model* to see how building a base is a necessary perquisite to injury free HIIT training. Otherwise known as "moderate pace," this zone runs between 70–80 percent of your MHR and is the pace you keep when you are going for a steady state easy or long run. You should be in this zone between faster-training sessions. This zone should encompass most your running volume (80–90 percent). Here are the three basics to building your base before you get out there and become a roaring roadster with no gas.

1. *Long steady distance (LSD):* LSD is where you build your aerobic base, which all distance races feed upon. When first incorporating these distances, they can be as low as 60 percent effort

for your body to get use to spending long periods of time on your feet. But eventually you want to get them up to 80 percent effort (but no higher! 80 percent is roughly the aerobic threshold; if you start to work harder, you are no longer working aerobically, thus not focusing on the goal of the workout). At first perform one LSD run every two weeks, and then once your body becomes accustomed to them, you can step it up to once per week if it does not hinder your performance for the rest of your weekly training. The distance of your LSD should be 20–30 percent of your total weekly mileage. So, if you are running sixty miles per week, then your LSD day should be twelve to eighteen miles. Higher mileage and frequency runners stay toward the 20 percent end, and lower total mileage and frequency runners use the 30 percent value. But make sure to take your time building up to that distance, increasing your mileage no more than 10 percent per week. Remember building up too fast only increases your chance of injury, and you cannot get faster when you're on the injured list.

Long Runs Should be 20%-30% of Your Weekly Mileage

2. *Hills for strength:* I know I said do not throw in intervals without a proper base first. However, hills offer you something speed intervals do not, strength. For your muscles to get stronger, they need to fight against a resistance (in this case gravity via going up a hill), not increase speed (two hundred meters on a track). It is resistance not speed that builds muscle, and for this reason, hills should be done during the middle to later stage of the base-building phase to increase strength so we are stronger once it is time to introduce speed workouts in order to blast through faster track intervals with a lower risk of injury. When starting hill repeats, begin with six to ten short and intense repeats lasting eight to ten seconds, adding one more repetition every week. After you reach fifteen repetitions, move up to four to eight repetitions of twenty- to thirty-second hills, at a calmer yet still fast pace. Build up to twelve repetitions, and then perform four to six repetitions of sixty- to ninety-second hill repeats at race pace, building up to eight to ten repetitions. The key points to remember with hills are the shorter the duration of the hill repeat, the steeper the hill and longer the rest.

　　　The hill training chart below will give you an idea of how hills can be performed depending on your goal. This chart is not to be taken as one size fits all advice, but as a guideline to build upon when devising your program. The shorter the hill, the faster you run the repeat and the longer the hill, the slower you run. Regardless of hill length, rest is relatively equal since the lack of speed on longer hills is made up by the time-under-tension running up a longer grade.

Hill Prescription

Length	Time	Intensity	Rest	Incline
Short	8-10 s	100%		12%-15%
Medium	20-30 s	95%-100%	60-180 s	8%-10%
Long	60-90 s	85%-95%		4%-6%

3. *Rest to rejuvenate and rebuild:* Although the final section of this book is titled "Rest and Recovery," I need to mention here that it is while we rest that our body becomes stronger. Resting gives our body and mind a chance to rejuvenate and replenish our energy stores while rebuilding broken down muscle tissues. Our mind also needs a break, mental fatigue and burnout occurs when we keep intensity elevated for too long without a rest day or longer

recovery period. Research has shown our mind needs to recover in the same manner as our body. So remember to wait forty-eight hours between all hard efforts (recovery and easy efforts are a part of training). It is the easiest part of getting faster; don't skip out on it.

Building a base is essential to endurance sports because that is the foundation of their strength. With that said, ball sports also benefit from base building prior to HIIT because it raises the anaerobic threshold, meaning athletes can compete longer before working aerobically and second, the low intensity repetitive stress is a good primer for the mechanical demands of HIIT. Yet, as important as base building is for endurance athletes, and the majority of their training should be spent in the aerobic zone, the majority of high-intensity sports training must focus on HIIT after establishing a base to become competitive.

Race Pace: Lactic threshold training has been used by runners for years. It is perhaps the most important form of training for getting yourself in race shape. With that said, we have learned through research that there are different forms of lactic threshold training depending on your goal's race distance and relative intensity. We must train differently to hit each goal. However, to see the best results, we should incorporate a mix of all three types of lactic threshold training into our routines.

During a race as the intensity increases, the amount of lactate accumulating in your muscles increases as well until it reaches the point where your muscles cannot clear out the lactate as fast it is building up, and you start to slow down, as discussed earlier. What we have come to learn is the rate at which lactate builds up in your muscles varies depending on the length and relative intensity of the race. The higher the intensity, the quicker lactate builds up. For that reason, it only makes sense to train your lactate threshold using different techniques depending on the nature of the lactate accumulation rate. It has also been decided by some in the field including myself to refer to lactic threshold training as race-pace training when referring to endurance sports, because as we move away from the typical "twenty minutes at threshold pace" and start to develop more individualized training programs for varying distances, we believe that the term "race-pace training" is better suited.

For our purposes let's break races distances and intensities into three different categories:

1. *Low-speed/high-volume:* These include races lasting between two and three hours.

2. *Moderate-speed/volume:* For races lasting between one and two hours.

3. *High-speed/low-volume:* For races lasting less than one hour (generally thirty to forty-five minutes).

Low-speed/high-volume: Races in this zone range from half marathons to marathons. The workout should last between forty and ninety minutes, increasing the time spent at race pace as you become more accustomed to it at shorter durations. Training at race pace is important especially for distances of such length because your body should become an efficiency monster at race pace if it is expected to hold it for such a long time.

Moderate-speed/volume: These races range from 10 miles to 20k. These workouts last between twenty and forty minutes at race pace.

High-speed/low-volume: These are your repeats for races 5–10k. While doing these, it is important to remember that they are not anaerobic repeats. They are still race-pace repeats for endurance races, and the pace should be equivalent to race pace, no faster. A good way to keep pace in check is to keep the work to rest ratio low such as 5:1 (work:rest). This will force runners to hold back, so they can make it through their entire workout. A good trick that will get your pace roughly in the correct training is to add five seconds per mile for every ten minutes over twenty minutes your workout plans on being. So, if you are running six-minute miles for a standard twenty-minute tempo run, then you would be running 6:10 miles for forty minutes (RunnersWorld.com). Note: This pace starts after a proper warm-up.

There are many benefits to training at race pace. It prepares our body to run at certain lactate levels, teaching us that racing in the discomfort zone is acceptable. The important thing to remember is volume not speed yields the best results during these workouts. We are not trying to enhance "launch time" (that is for a different workout), but we are trying to enhance efficiency at race pace. Don't bother training for your sprint to the finish if you have not trained at race pace first, so you can get there.

Race Pace Training is About Time Spent Training at Race Pace, Not Faster

VO2max (Maximum effort/VO2max threshold pace): Working in this zone is not for the faint of heart. It involves getting up to 98 percent of your MHR for brief amounts of time (note: the whole interval is not at 98 percent MHR). These intervals are done for no longer than five minutes without a break. The point of VO_2max training is to increase your ability to get oxygen to the working muscles. To give you an example of how hard the pace is, the effort is one that you cannot maintain running for more than two miles. The pace is 85–95 percent VO_2max (92–98 percent MHR) or ten to thirty seconds faster per mile than your 5k-race pace.

Repetition Pace (sprint repetition): This zone is short and brutal. It is performed faster/harder than your VO_2max pace; although it does increase VO_2max, it does not develop it as effectively as performing VO_2max intervals. Repetitions improve your races by developing your running economy and enhancing your speed. Each repetition should be performed at 95–100 percent MHR, in other words, all out for short periods. Running sprints are generally shorter than two hundred meters.

The Higher the Intensity, the Less Time We Need Training at That Intensity

Type of Training	Percent of Training Volume	Percent of Max Heart Rate	Purpose of Activity
Aerobic	80%-90% (90% for base building)	50%-80%	Improve fat utilization.
Race Pace	10%	80%-90%	Become more efficient at race pace.
VO₂max Intervals	7%	92%-98% (Potentially peaking at 98% for moments)	Increase VO₂max.
Sprint Repetitions	3%	95%-100%	Increase running efficiency and speed.

As runners, we have all become so amped up in the weeks leading up to a race that we decide to take our training up a notch and push ourselves a little harder than we should. We become so focused on hitting our goal time or beating a buddy in an upcoming race that we start running faster every time we head out the door for a training run only to get to race day and finish with a less than stellar performance. After the race, you'll begin to ask yourself questions like, "Why did this happen? I trained harder than I ever trained before, where did I go wrong?" Then you may realize the answer is obvious. In retrospect, you see that you had been training too fast.

There is a difference between training too fast and training too hard. By training faster, we must pick up the pace, but to train harder, you can also increase your volume, add more hills, decrease your rest interval, or up your frequency. These are the variables that a runner should focus on when deciding to up his intensity.

Distance running is an aerobic sport, relying mainly on fat as fuel. Although the other energy systems contribute to energy production during a run, our fat stores provide more energy than we would need for most endurance activities (even for an elite marathoner). This is because evolution made us "fat efficient."

Evolution Made Us Efficient at Burning Fat, Training Improves That Gift

The problem with increasing training pace is that you will likely enter the anaerobic zone (without oxygen). Your anaerobic gateway begins at 80 percent max heart rate (MHR). Once you are here, you are no longer primarily focusing on enhancing your body's ability to use fat as fuel. Consequently, come race day your body is less efficient at using its primary endurance fuel source (fat) than it was prior to your increased training intensity because it has become accustomed to burning a higher percentage of carbohydrates as fuel, whereas a distance race relies predominantly on fat as fuel. We can slightly raise our max heart rate with training; however, our main benefit for fat utilization is elevating the anaerobic threshold, so we can run at higher intensities aerobically with fat as our main fuel source. This allows athletes to run at a faster pace before fatigue sets in, causing our pace to diminish. We are in essence raising the bar.

Working on your base, under 80 percent max heart rate, increases your VO₂max up to 20 percent and endurance up to 10,000 percent! But when we get into race-pace training, we should only expect an increase of up to 3 percent (Finke and Finke 2004). Think of race-pace training as sharpening the blade. Sharpening the blade is useless if you did not take the time to fortify the metal making it strong enough to withstand the stress of the initial strike.

Most of an Endurance Athlete's Progress Occurs Below the Ventilatory Threshold

A useful tip for while you're out on a run to ensure you are working in the aerobic zone is reciting the pledge of allegiance. If you can say it without gasping for air, then you are working aerobically.

Notice how large the portion dedicated to aerobic training is in the chart below. Athletes need to spend more time training aerobically prior to engaging in anaerobic metabolic conditioning. This does two things, first it enhances our ability to use fat as fuel, and second it raises the bar at which we enter anaerobic metabolism (it holds off heavy breathing).

Ideal Distance Runner Training Volume Distribution

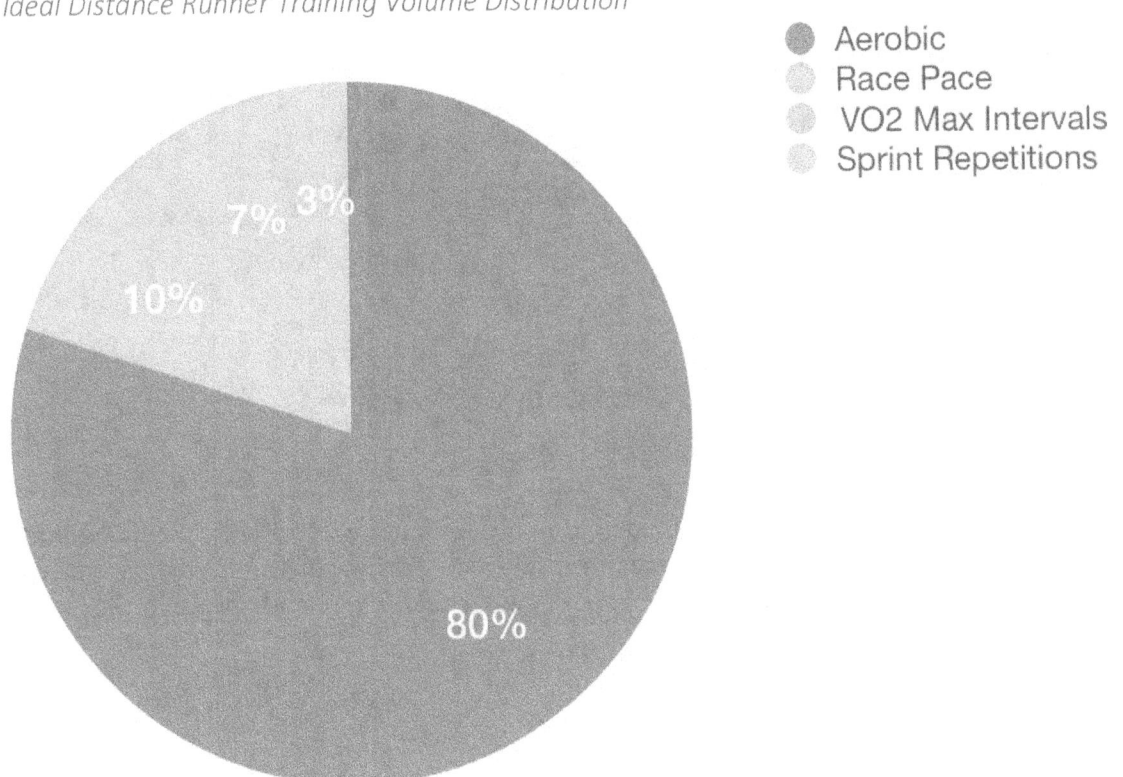

I know it can be difficult to distinguish between the shades in this pie chart, but *Metabolic Training for Distance Runners' Volume Breakdown* is the corresponding table. The big take away here is how aerobic training consumes the majority of the chart for distance runners.

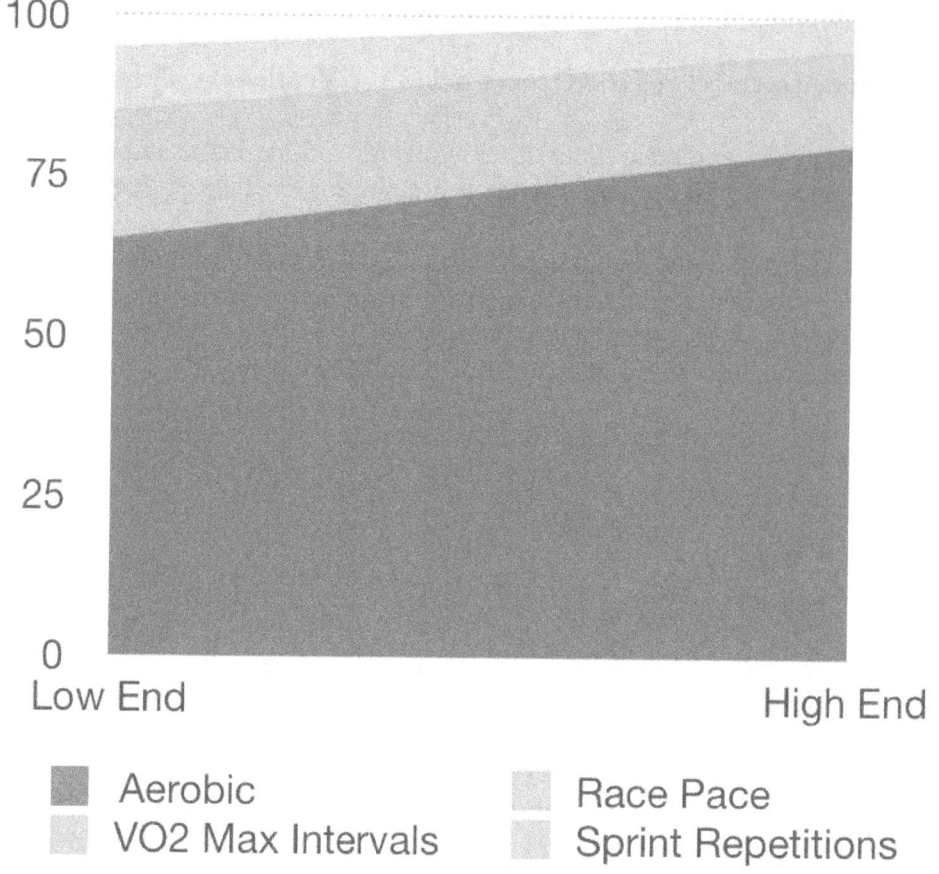

Muscle Fiber Activation Thresholds by Heart Rate

■ Aerobic	■ Race Pace
■ VO2 Max Intervals	■ Sprint Repetitions

This chart shows you the threshold range during which muscle fibers enter a new training stimulus. Once heart rate hits the athlete's individual threshold within a given range, low-end or high-end, they are focusing on training the focus listed above (aerobic, ventilatory threshold, VO_2max intervals, repetitions sprints).

Rest and Recovery

The Importance of Rest and Sleep for Physical Improvement

As we know from previous chapters, your body needs its recovery time as it needs its periods of activity. Without it, your body will eventually go into a state of overtraining, and your performance will steadily decline.

With that said, the most important form of rest is sleep. During non-rapid eye movement (NREM), specifically N3 (the third stage of NREM sleep), your body is undergoing its major repairs. While sleeping, our body is acting as a canvas to rebuild. As you sleep, your body enters a catabolic (nonmuscle building and performance enhancing) state that if properly nourished can be transformed into an anabolic muscle-building and performance-enhancing playground. When properly fueled with slow-acting casein protein before going to bed, your body undergoes improved protein synthesis. This paired with heightened levels of growth hormone naturally occurring while sleeping lead to an anabolic holiday. If you do not get the most out of these two variables, you are truly missing out on athletic gains.

What happens during N3, the restorative and rebuilding stage of sleep:

1. Muscles relax
2. Breathing slows and blood pressure drops
3. Muscle growth and repair
4. Growth hormone release
5. Energy restoration

Additionally, when your body lacks sleep, your neuromuscular connections are not as quick or firing at their best, and your energy levels are down the toilet. Resulting in less than superb workouts when you are supposed to be working intensely. On top of that, it is not only the quantity of sleep that matters but the quality. Our body responds better to sleep between 11:00 p.m. and 7:00 a.m. than 2:00 a.m. and 10:00 a.m. because the body is used to a cycle based on daylight over the past thousands of years. Our quality of sleep is also negatively affected by electronics. Their bright displays mimic sunlight to our brain, hindering our ability to fall asleep after using them at night.

Our Best Sleep Generally Occurs from 11:00 PM – 7:00 AM

Adequate sleep is vital to any athlete's success regardless of his or her discipline. It is recommended that athletes get at least eight hours of sleep per night, so their bodies can properly repair and re-energize for the workouts ahead. Here are four quick tips to get to sleep quicker and stay asleep longer.

1. *No internet or TV:* Studies show that people who use handheld devices or watch TV while in bed take an extra thirty to sixty minutes trying to fall asleep. Although blue screens reduce light activating the brain, we are still exciting our brain by taking in new information when we should be relaxing. If you need something to make you tired, read the most boring book you can find. Hopefully I am not providing that book, but if so, you're welcome.

2. *Cut back on late-night exercise:* People who exercise within two to three hours of trying to fall asleep have a much harder time doing so than people who exercise earlier in the day.

3. *Dark room:* We sleep at night for a reason—it is easier to fall asleep and stay asleep when you are in a dark room. With that said, make sure you have blackout shades over your windows and all light-emitting, electronic devices off in your room.

4. *Avoid simple sugars:* Simple sugars go to your bloodstream fast, giving you readily available energy quick. This is not something you want when you are trying to sleep.

Overall, if you have a night or two per week of little sleep (less than eight hours), it is not going to make or break your workouts. But if you are missing more than that on a regular basis, you can put your body into a state of overtraining. So, squeeze the most out of your workouts, and get plenty of rest and sleep at night.

Lack of Sleep has a Similar Consequence as Overtraining

We've all been there. We had the game of our lives on Saturday morning, and then on Sunday night, it hurts to move our back. Or we smash our old PR in a race on Saturday morning and can't walk down the stairs on Monday. Sometimes we say to ourselves, "Is it really worth being so sore for days after my competition that I can barely walk?"

Obviously, you're expecting me to say yes. It always hurts more to look back and know you did not have the guts to compete than it does to have gone out there and ran your body to the junkyard, and yes, that is what I am saying. Don't worry though, I do have good news. There is a way to get your body to recover faster, so you're not lingering around your living room days after your competition. The simple solution is keep moving! Lightly, of course.

The worst thing you can do for your body after you have broken it down is lie in bed and sleep all day. That hurting feeling in your muscles is part of your body's natural-healing process. It is trying to get nutrient- and oxygen-rich blood to its aching muscles, so it can heal faster, and we all know there is not a lot of blood flow when you're sitting around all day. So what do you do?

Move! Go for a light walk, jog, ride, or swim. Get your body up and moving, so it can get blood flowing to the muscles. The additional blood flow delivers nutrients to the muscles as well as helps clear lactic acid and recover from Delayed Onset Muscle Soreness (DOMS). Now, I am not talking about anything intense. Staying in the 50–70 percent max heart range is great. No need to go any higher. The point of this light activity is not to get a workout (we do not want further muscle breakdown at this point); it is simply to speed up the healing process that our body does naturally. The enhanced blood flow refuels and repairs broken-down connective tissue (muscles, tendons, and ligaments).

Light Activity Speeds Recovery

Also, light stretching and self-myofascial release (pressure point therapy applied to oneself) can be beneficial after a competition. Remember to perform your stretches lightly; we don't want to further tear already broken-down muscle tissue. Use this tip next time you're sore and think the best remedy is popcorn and a movie in bed all day, and I guarantee you'll be back on the track in no time.

Note: I know you are all intelligent people, you would not be reading a book like this if you were not, but now is a good time for me to remind you to see a medical doctor if you are experiencing pain. I am not a medical doctor.

We have all been there, and if you haven't, you most likely will be at some point, and no, I'm not talking about Disney World. I'm talking about getting injured. Athletic injuries can happen for many reasons, either acute (suddenly like an ankle sprain or ACL tear) or chronic (such as runner's knee or low back pain). Although even some acute injuries are a result of a chronic buildup over time, that is, your ankle sprained because you have a weak ankle.

Injuries can be a real downer. You see everyone else around you competing with such ease, yet you're stuck either doing prone hamstring curls with a 3 lb. ankle weight or sitting at home on your coach icing your leg for twenty minutes, three times per day. The purpose of this chapter is not to help speedup the healing process physiologically but rather psychologically. Here is a short list to help you cope with your athletic injury so your time on the sidelines isn't more painful than your Monday 5:30 a.m. workout.

1. Realization: The first step in dealing with an athletic injury is realizing you have one. Running around on a sore ankle is not going to help it heal faster, nor is bench pressing with pain in your rotator cuff. There is a difference between discomfort from an intense workout and pain from an injury. Realize the difference, and admit to yourself when it's the later.

2. Research: After you have realized you have an injury and not just a little DOMS from your last workout, it's time to figure out what went wrong. There are numerous things that can be wrong in one area. This is not the time to assume that since your buddy had runner's knee that you have runner's knee because your knee hurts too. Speak with a qualified sports-medicine doctor to see what is wrong and figure out what to do next.

3. Remember and Repeat: Remember what the sports-medicine specialist told you, and repeat the exercises you were instructed to perform. This is most people's downfall with recovery. They realize they have an injury and seek help, but when they should do something to fix it, they drop the ball. Listen to your medical doctor; they are the professionals for a reason. Alternatively, if you can't seem to stick through with it on your own, hire a corrective-exercise specialist to help you through.

4. Removal: Temptation can ruin a lot of things. Including athletic careers. If you're the type of person who cannot resist to jump back in the game before you're fully healed, then the last thing you want to be doing is placing yourself in that situation. If you know you can't resist temptation, then stay away from it.

5. Reminisce: Eventually even though you are doing all the right steps, you are going to be upset or even angry that healing is such a slow process, which it can be. When this happens, start reminiscing about all you have accomplished until the injury and how good you will feel once the injury has been resolved. Because you will get there again!

6. Reintroduce and Rebuild: When it is finally time to start introducing old exercises and workouts to your routine, remember you have been performing prone leg curls or ankle mobility only for the past month or more, and now is not the time to test your 1RM dead lift or jump in a 5k. Start easy, and work your way up. The confidence booster from finishing an easy workout will be more satisfying than trying to do what you could before the injury, and you will not only be disappointing yourself because you are not ready but also getting reinjured.

Now that you know the R method of coping with athletic injury, please use it in its entirety. Not only because it will help you deal with being on the sidelines and speed up the process, but because being proactive in getting yourself back on the field, court, or track is always better than sitting there waiting for a miracle.

1. Realization
2. Research
3. Remember & Repeat
4. Removal
5. Reminisce
6. Reintroduce
7. Rebuild

The dreaded muscle cramp is every athlete's nightmare. At some point in your career, chances are you have encountered a muscle cramp, and chances are it was not pleasant. What causes a muscle cramp is still uncertain, but scientists have made assumptions. One assumption, which is also the most famous one, is muscle cramps are a result of dehydration, an electrolyte imbalance. Studies, however, have shown that people who experience cramps have the same electrolyte levels as people who do not experience cramps. Furthermore, when you experience a cramp, you are typically more hydrated than people who do not experience cramps. Therefore, that theory has more than its fair share of holes.

What is it then that causes muscle cramps during physical activity? Another and more reliable theory supporting the reasoning behind muscle cramps is a misfiring of the muscles during physical activity because of the muscle spindle reflex (contracts muscles) and the Golgi tendon organ reflex (relaxes muscles). Research suggests that muscle cramps occur when alpha motor neurons (electric nerve impulses causing your muscles to contract) are firing when they shouldn't due to miscommunication with the muscle spindle reflex and the Golgi tendon organ reflex. What is happening is the muscle spindle reflex is causing the muscle to contract, and the Golgi tendon organ reflex is being inhibited, causing the painful tightening of the muscle that occurs during a muscle cramp. This is occurring because the muscles are fatigued, and just like your brain, when your muscles are fatigued, they make mistakes.

This theory gives a much better explanation of what may cause a muscle cramp. Now that you know what may be causing your muscles to cramp, you need to know how to avoid muscle cramps. Since electrolytes and hydration are most likely not to blame, chances are they will not solve the problem either. Therefore, the solution must be located somewhere within the tension of the muscles. For that reason, it is believed that a period of stretching (at least eight to twelve seconds allowing the Golgi tendon organ reflex to kick in and an additional twenty to sixty seconds to relax the muscles) will be your best bet at fighting muscle cramps. Stretching is resetting the muscle to its proper level of tension. If stretching does not help, then try applying pressure to the area and maintaining that pressure for one minute. Applying pressure to an overactive muscle sends a signal similar to stretching. I prefer a lacrosse ball or tennis ball to target the area. If the area is not tender, then there is no need to apply pressure.

Stretching and Pressure Point Therapy Relieves Muscle Cramps

Running is primarily a pulling and not a pushing movement and is composed of three phases: push-off, recovery from push-off, and landing. The hip's hyperextensors pull you forward as one foot "claws" at the ground by your plantar flexors (push-off), and then the leg tucks in high by your gluteus maximus (recovery from push-off), swings forward, and extends outward as it prepares for its next step (landing).

During a single step of a stride, your leg is extended in front of your torso by your hip flexors while your knee is being extended by your quads. Once your foot contacts the ground, it claws back as you extend your hips using your gluteus maximus and hamstrings. Note, because your knee is almost fully extended as it goes into landing, it cannot further extend to launch you forward like one might imagine but rather relies on the hip hyperextensors to do the heavy work. Sometimes this cycle can be interrupted by muscle imbalances and poor arthrokinematics (joint dysfunctions). The most common case being tight hip flexors (iliopsoas) from sitting in chairs all day. Whether it is work, driving, or even our bike, being in a seated position causes our hip flexors to shorten over time. In turn, this causes our gluteus maximus to inhibit or weaken, due to reciprocal inhibition, as one muscle activates or shortens, its opposing muscle must lengthen. As runners reach faster speeds, their gluteus maximus is supposed to contribute more toward hip hyperextension. However, because our gluteus maximus is weakened, it causes our hamstrings, which produce hip hyperextension at slower speeds and assist during faster speeds, to overcompensate. This is called synergistic dominance. Synergistic dominance of our hamstrings is the reason many runners have tight hamstrings. The hamstrings are working overtime to make up for our gluteus maximus, becoming tight, fatigued, and prone to injury.

Weak Glutes & Core as Well as Tight Hip Flexors & Hamstrings Arise from Sitting

This dilemma goes further because the erector spinae muscles in our low back act as a stabilizer and support the body while the prime movers are responsible for locomotion and other larger movements. The erector spinae is also working overtime to assist the hamstrings in doing the gluteus maximus' job. This causes our erector spinae to shorten, resulting in reciprocal inhibition of our rectus abdominals (abs). So we are stuck with weak abs, and our pelvis undergoes what is known as an anterior tilt, rocking forward, or lower-crossed syndrome, tilted to the rear. This in turn shortens our stride. When our pelvis is rocked forward, it is typically because of the following: tight erector spinae, weak gluteus maximus, weak abdominals, tight iliopsoas. This situation hinders us from being able to lift our leg high during hip flexion and thus restrains it from covering as much ground as possible during each stride. Seeing how running pace is the product of stride length (force) times stride frequency (turnover), we now have a slower pace because frequency typically remains constant (160–180 steps per minute depending on our running ability, that is, beginner versus elite), but our stride length is covering less distance.

How do we fix the problem? Gluteus Maximus activation re-educates the gluteus maximus (big butt muscle) to fire properly with the hamstrings. Do this by performing Romanian dead lifts, good mornings, and high step-ups. Also, inhibit the hip flexors using self-myofascial release (SMR) such as a foam roller, lacrosse ball, manual therapy, or static stretch. The combination of these two strategies will strengthen weak muscles and relax overactive muscles. After a few weeks, your body will begin working in sync, and you will see an improvement in your performance.

Tight
Erector
Spinae

Weak
Abdominal

Weak
Gluteus
Maxiums

Tight
Iliopsoas

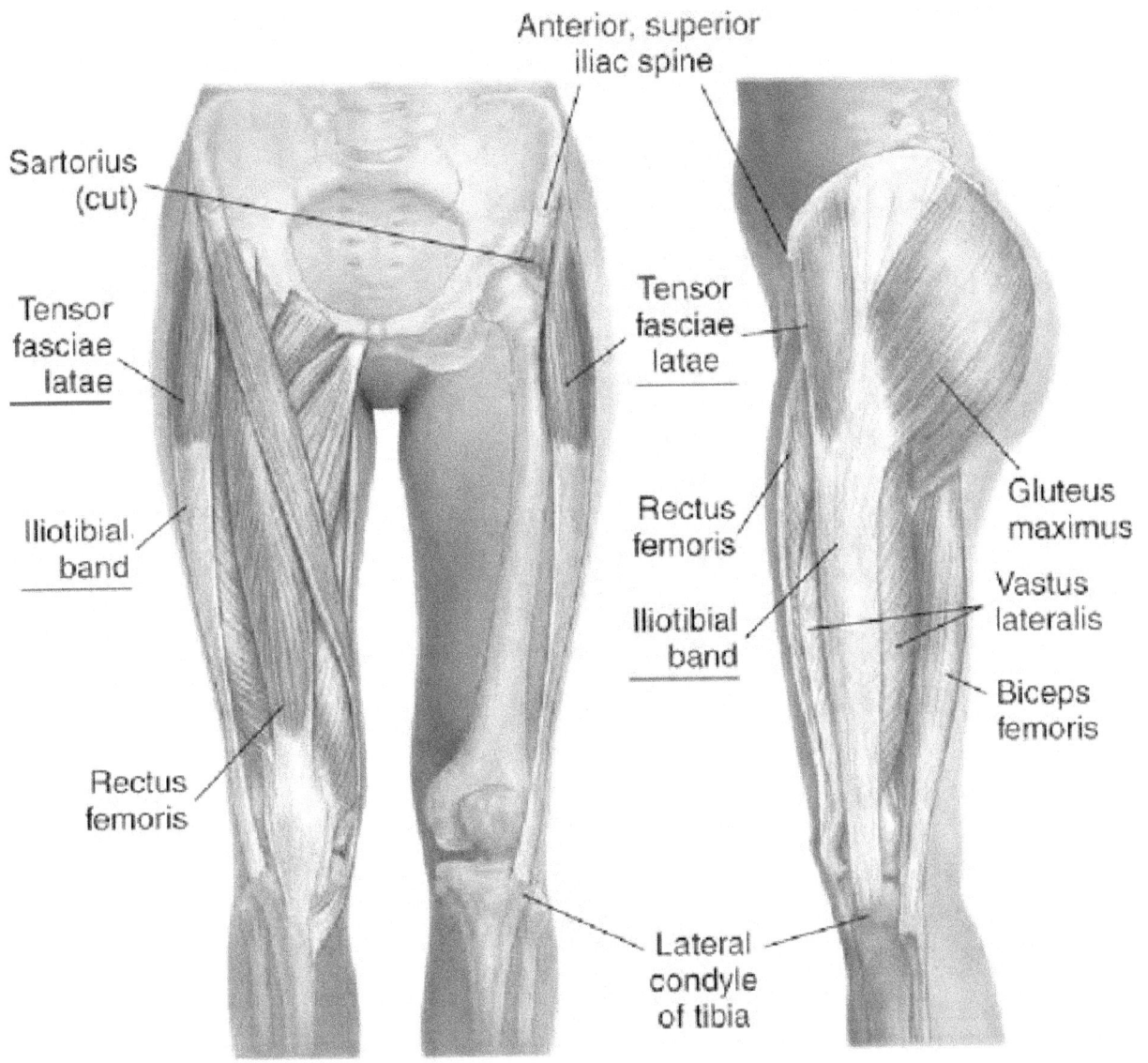

Anterior, superior
iliac spine

Sartorius
(cut)

Tensor
fasciae
latae

Iliotibial
band

Rectus
femoris

Tensor
fasciae
latae

Rectus
femoris

Iliotibial
band

Lateral
condyle
of tibia

Gluteus
maximus

Vastus
lateralis

Biceps
femoris

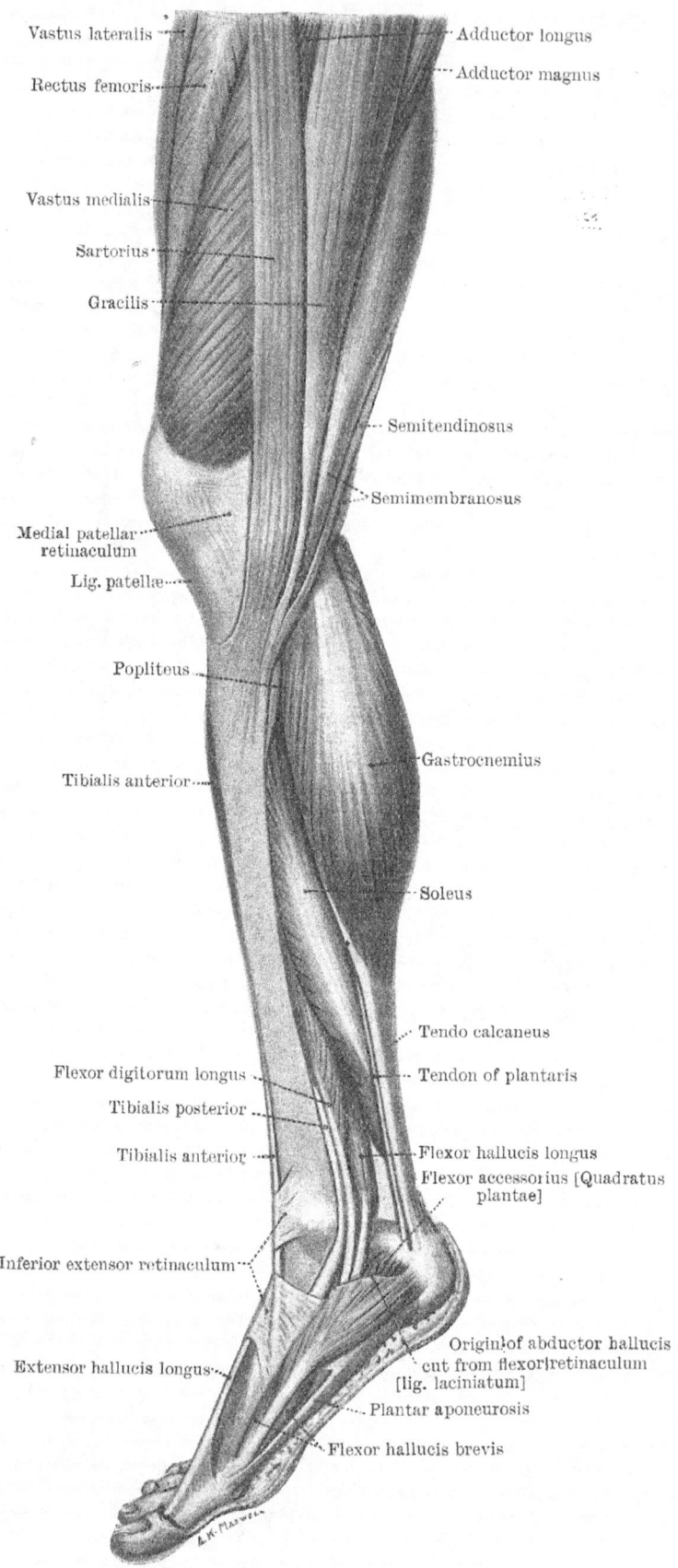

Vastus lateralis

Rectus femoris

Vastus medialis

Sartorius

Gracilis

Medial patellar retinaculum

Lig. patellæ

Popliteus

Tibialis anterior

Flexor digitorum longus

Tibialis posterior

Tibialis anterior

Inferior extensor retinaculum

Extensor hallucis longus

Adductor longus

Adductor magnus

Semitendinosus

Semimembranosus

Gastrocnemius

Soleus

Tendo calcaneus

Tendon of plantaris

Flexor hallucis longus

Flexor accessorius [Quadratus plantae]

Origin of abductor hallucis cut from flexor retinaculum [lig. laciniatum]

Plantar aponeurosis

Flexor hallucis brevis

Knowing all this, sometimes when we see hooves in the dirt, it may be a zebra. What I mean by this is, don't always go with the textbook scenario. Just because hoof prints are typically from horses, don't forget zebras are out there too. Far too often new coaches will blurt out the previous scenario without performing a proper assessment to determine if it's the case.

Squatting is one of the primary exercises athletes perform to improve performance, yet when working with new athletes I tend to see one common dysfunction, an excessive forward lean with heels elevated. Although an excessive forward lean can be caused by lower-crossed syndrome (tight hip flexors and hamstrings and inhibited abdominals and glutes), I began to notice a recurring trend where their heels were also leaving the ground.

After doing some research, I stumbled across a few findings that suggest a lack of ankle mobility can be more to do with an excessive forward lean while squatting, specifically a lack of dorsiflexion due to a weak anterior tibialis (front of shin) and tight Gastrocnemius (calf). This lack of mobility in the ankle limits the hip's ability to fully extend while walking and running which overtime causes an anterior tilt of the pelvis. This tilt forward and down (picture pouring a bowl of cereal onto the ground in front of you from your pelvis) leads to a shorted hipflexor and an over lengthened and taut hamstring.

Although similar to lower crossed syndrome, it is different since the hamstring is lengthened and taut rather than shortened and overactive. This means the tension is not a result of the hamstring outperforming the glutes, but rather the ankle causing restricted motion and an anterior tilt of the pelvis. Tightness is a sensation, not a symptom and we tend to mistake the sensation of taut muscles as tight muscles. Our taut hamstrings are a result of tight calfs pulling and lengthening the hamstrings. Knowing this, we should not treat our hamstrings as tight shortened muscles, but rather taut lengthened muscles.

Tightness is a Sensation, Muscles May be Short & Contracted or Lengthened and Taut

For this reason, it must be treated differently by first rolling your foot over a golf ball for one minute, then rolling a lacrosse ball over your peroneals (side of your lower leg), both hemispheres of your Gastrocnemius (left and right sides of your calf), rolling on a lacrosse ball on the proximal end (directly under your butt cheek) of your hamstring to reduce the taut nature of the hip and stretching your hip flexors.

Upon completing these preparatory exercises, I would recommend glute bridges and performing anterior tibialis strengthening exercises such as forward leans and prone ankle dorsi flexion (lie on the floor in the prone position and place a mini band around both feet, then flex one foot towards your shin) to isolated the weak muscles. Followed by forefoot elevated overhead squats with a PVC pipe where the balls of your feet are elevated on small plates, as well as posterior chain squats on a TRX to integrate all the movements at once.

Of course, there is more you can do for this situation, but I am a firm believer in providing enough to get started so it is not overwhelming, then adding more as you go. Also, remember that every situation is unique, and you are best meeting with a professional to determine what is truly happening.

Here are the exercises laid out for you as a workout.

Inhibit

2. Roll with a golf ball; plantar fascia (1 min)
3. Roll with a lacrosse ball; lateral and medial gastrocnemius and proximal attachment of hamstrings (3 min)
4. Foam roll peroneals (3 min)
5. Stretch hip flexors (1 min)

Isolate

1. Forward leans (1 x 15)
2. Glute bridges (1 x 15)
3. Prone mini band ankle dorsiflexion (1 x 15)

Integrate

4. PVC forefoot elevated overhead squat (2 x 8)
5. Posterior chain squat TRX squats (1 x 8)

The Spine and the Foot, One in the Same

People often seek me out with low back issues, describing to me the sensations they are feeling in their low back while placing their hands on the quadratus lumborum (low back) and rubbing the area, then when I ask them to take off their shoes they look at me weird.

We have the tendency to place blame for pain on the area that is in discomfort, when the majority of our dysfunctions begin somewhere else. As bipedal animals, our first point of contact with the outside world is through our feet. This is why I have clients take off their shoes during an assessment (I later assess them wearing shoes to determine if the shoe is the culprit). With that said, pain and discomfort we experience in our back is commonly influenced by our feet's effect on posture.

When examining posture, I first look to see if a client's feet are externally rotated (supination), neutral, or pronated (arch caves-in). If I see a client's foot is over-pronating, then I generally assume their same side psoas and adductors will be short and tight. This will result in a weak glute and sometimes lower crossed syndrome. Another give away of overpronation is a bunion on the big toe.

If when I examine a client's feet and I see their foot externally rotating or supinating, then I know their vastus lateralis (outside of thigh) is strong. Knowing this, if the outside of their leg is strong, the inside will most likely be weak, so I check for weak adductors. Since they're walking on the outside of their foot, their same side gluteus maximus muscle will generally be shortened and tight as will their quadratus lumborum. This is more often than not the result of their back pain, and I generally provide corrective exercise to remedy their foot external rotation and their back pain alleviates with time.

These corrective exercise strategies vary from person to person, but I mostly examine their arch and make adjustments observing how those adjustments affect the thoracolumbar-pelvic canister (entire torso, shoulders to hips). The foot can be thought of like your spine, they are both designed to have natural curvatures and if they are lacking these curvatures, issues arise.

Upon manipulating a client's arch, if there is an improvement, I will recommend manual therapy for their lower leg as well as arch building exercises such as towel scrunches. Once their posture is back on track, we can begin strengthening and inhibiting the respective areas in the hips and back.

Our feet's impact on our low back is another example of how our problems sometimes reside outside of our pain. For this reason, it is important we take note of different walking patterns, shoes, sleeping patterns, chairs, and other things of that nature in order to gain more detail into injuries.

The rotator cuff muscles (supraspinatus, infraspinatus, subscapularis, and teres minor) and shoulder girdle (clavicle and scapula bones) should not be examined without understanding the hip and ankle complex. It is a common belief in my field that many shoulder injuries excluding blunt trauma (a sudden hit) begin at the ankle or hip, which in turn limits motion and control of the shoulder girdle, thus impacting the rotator cuff and connecting glenohumeral joint.

The Rotator Cuff Muscles

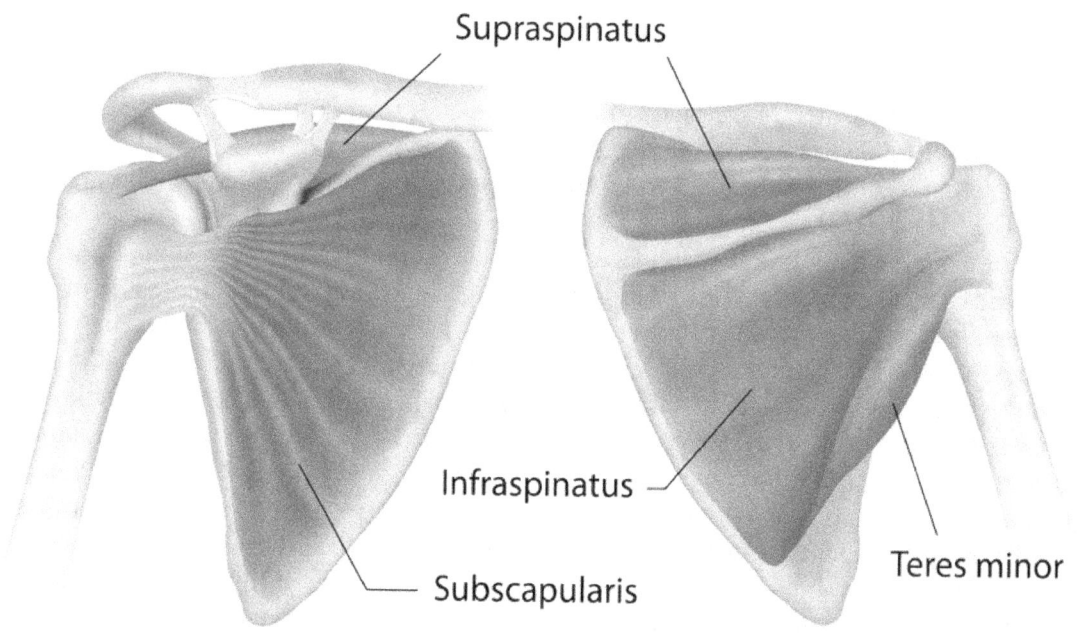

Anterior view   **Posterior view**

During hip extension, which is movement performed throughout the day, the scapula retracts and enhances shoulder flexion on the same side. The opposite is true for hip flexion; the scapula protracts and enhances shoulder extension. Similar scenarios exist for hip adduction and scapula adduction on the same side. Relationships between the hips such as these are why many shoulder impingement injuries stem from poor posture. An example is excessive forward leaning. As you lean forward, the scapula protracts and the acromion process pinches in the glenoid fossa, leading to shoulder impingement.

If we want to remedy shoulder injuries, we need to examine hip and ankle motion. We examine the ankle because of its role in hip mobility. With that said, plenty of injuries affecting the shoulder originated at the shoulder joint. These injuries can often be explained through lack of thoracic, scapula, and clavicular mobility, as well as a buildup of scar tissue or dehydrated fascia limiting the scapula's ability to glide over the thoracic spine properly. Dehydrated fascia is simply fascia that is less mobile because it has been less mobile. It's one of those use it or lose it things. If we are immobile in a joint for as little as 24 hours, we begin building what Dr. Gill Hedley refers to as "fuzz." Fuzz is a thickening of connective tissue limiting mobility. Fuzz is not a good thing and can be remedied through manual therapy such as massage and movement drills.

When examining the shoulder joint, I generally look for scapula mobility over the thoracic spine. If there is a scapula restriction and manually assisting the scapula in movement as the arm goes through a full range of motion helps, then the scapula may be the culprit, but if there is still discomfort or dysfunction when manually assisting in scapula motion, then I will look to the glenohumeral and elbow joint for restrictions. Beyond that, I assess how the hips, ankles, and spine react as the arm goes through a full range of motion.

Another common issue in the rotator cuff is an anterior positioning of the humorous in the glenoid fossa (shoulder joint) causing impingement. An overactive latissimus dorsi and teres major can be pulling the humorous anteriorly (forward) if the subscapularis is too weak to keep the joint in its proper position.

There are countless exercises for treating these dysfunctions, but with so much more going on for the shoulder than the hip, I feel a proper biometric analysis by a professional should be performed. With that said, one exercise that I have made a staple of my workouts is a modified Lawnmower Twist or dumbbell pullback into spinal extension with a slight twist of the spine towards the forward knee (see the pictures on the next two pages). I first saw the exercise performed by Chuck Wolf, and I have seen tremendous results as a general hip, spine, and shoulder mobility drill bringing the entire system into sync.

Walking away from this, the key takeaway is movement is unbelievably integrated. Isolated exercises have their place in immediate acute physical therapy but should be replaced by integrated movement patterns as soon as the body is ready. Most chronic injuries have a foundation in areas foreign to the pain and we must integrate whole body movements in order to correct posture and gait and keep the dysfunction from returning.

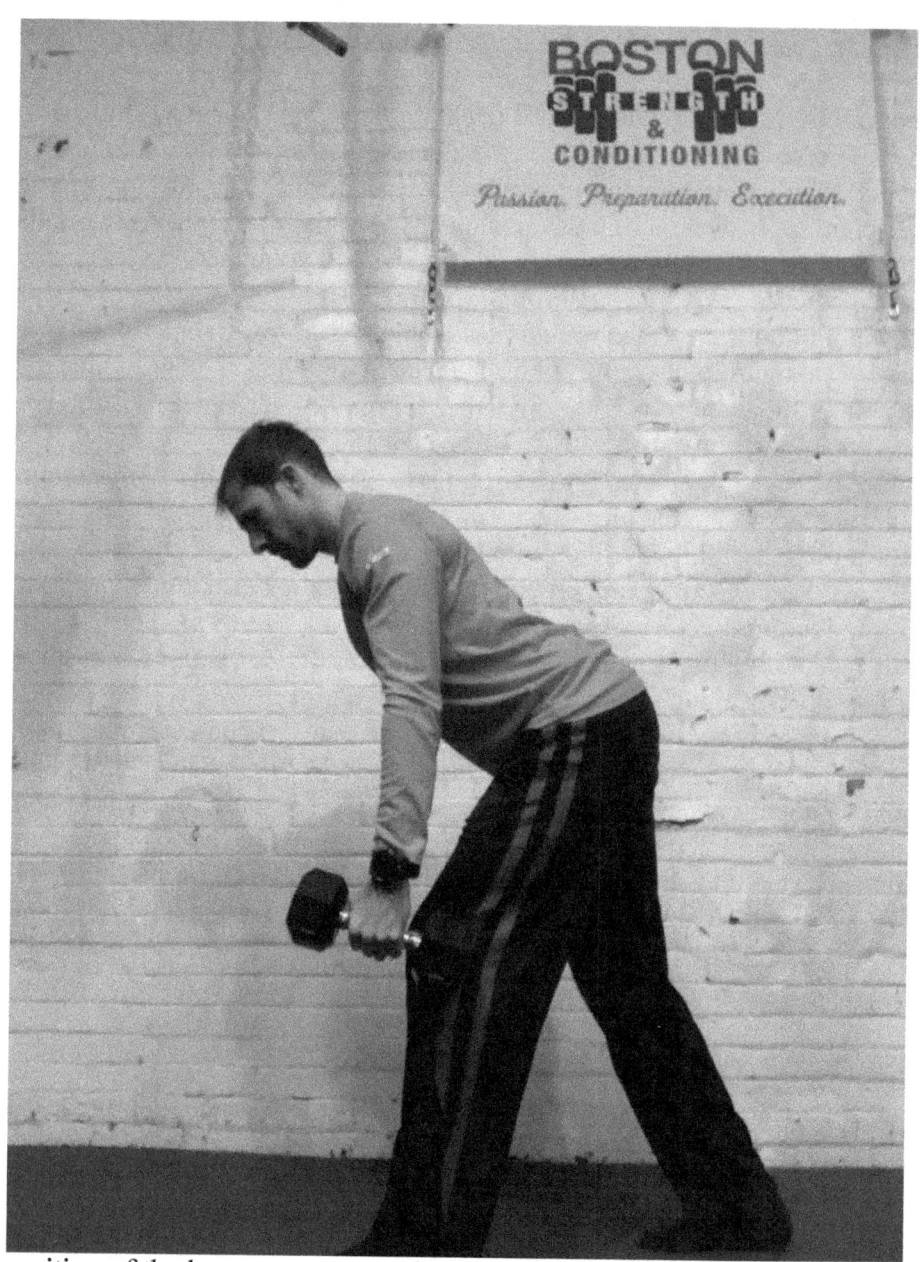

(Starting position of the lawnmower, note the neutral spine, flexion is occurring at the hips).

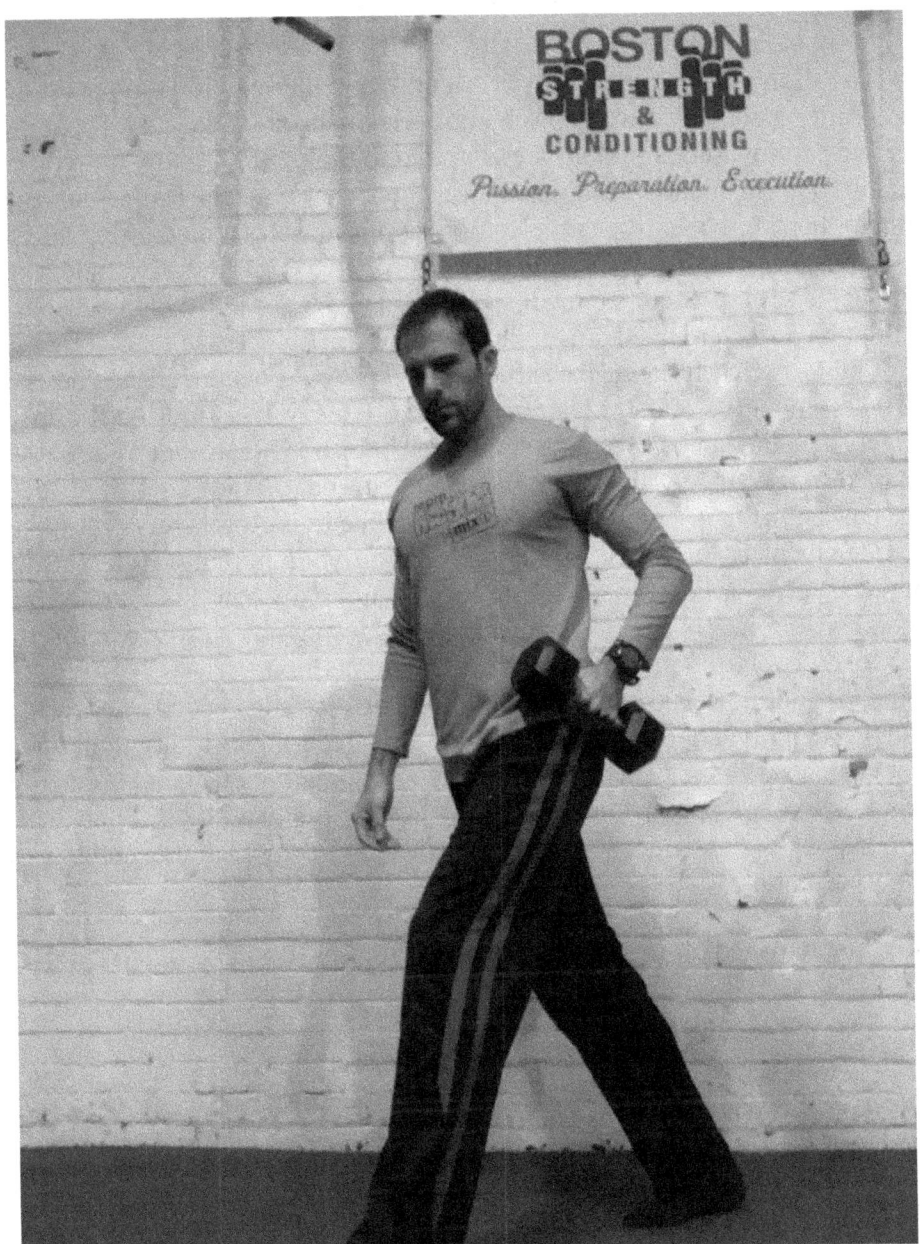

(Ending position of the lawnmower, belly button points towards lead leg's mid-thigh).

It happens all the time. An athlete starts a new training regimen with great results only to become injured after a couple of weeks. Why does this happen? If you are performing well and your muscles and cardiovascular system are adapting to the program, how did you get hurt? The answer is tendons and ligaments. Tendons and ligaments are noncontractile filaments that attach muscle to bone or bone to bone, respectively. While your muscles are enduring all the benefits of a vast blood supply and thus oxygen and nutrient supply, ensuring an efficient and adequate adaptation to the stresses of exercise, tendons and ligaments are left with a much lesser amount of blood resulting in a slower adaptation and healing process.

What's more is that because the structural breakdown occurring in your body takes so long, it has an accumulative effect. Meaning, if you do heavy legs on Monday and hard sprints on Thursday, your metabolic system may have been prepared for it, but your structural system may still be in recovery mode; thus your body will be put further back into recovery mode, meaning your chances of injury go up along with a decline in performance.

Consequently, it is important to keep an eye on your training cycle and listen to your body, so you know when it is acceptable to keep pushing and when it is time to back off. Over-reaching is good when it is systematically planned but be sure not to over-reach for too long and to leave plenty of recovery time for tapering prior to competition.

This means your muscles are adapting and feel great while becoming accustomed to their new workloads while your tendons and ligaments are on the brink of injury until one day they simply cannot keep up with the demands of training and something tears. Although we know better than to work through pain, nature did not give us the best warning single when something bad is about to happen to our tendons and ligaments. This is why planning and tracking all of your workouts is essential.

Muscles Have Better Access to Nutrients and Oxygen than Ligaments and Tendons

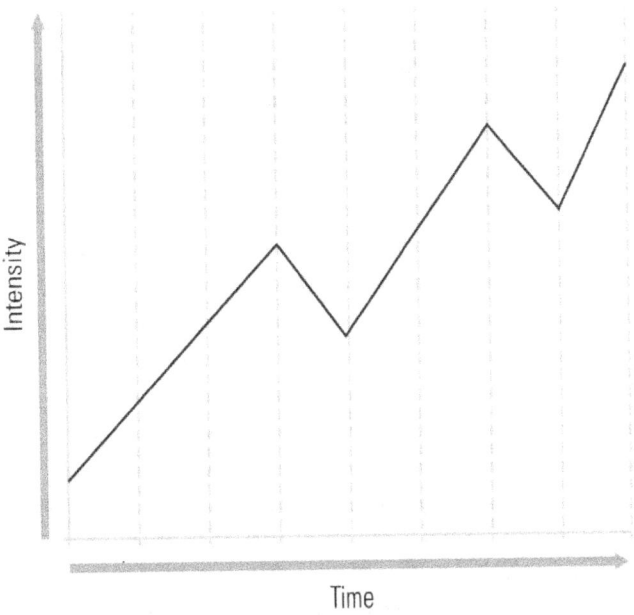

We Need Periods of Reduced Intensity After High Intensity to Adapt and Improve

What does this all mean to the athlete? Back off! Don't forget to take at least one day of complete rest every week, a "down week" or "unload week" every three to four weeks to allow your body to fully recuperate, and one to two weeks completely off every twelve to sixteen weeks. Yes, there are athletes who never take days off and avoid injury, but these athletes typically perform the same moderate-intensity workouts day after day. Moreover, research has proven repeatedly that varying intensity, that is, alternating easy and hard days, will stress the athlete's body in a manner that will yield better results. Remember, we are training to be excellent, not mediocre. Easy and off days are part of training towards excellence.

Your body is not designed to give you a whole lot of warning signs when a tendon or ligament is about to go, except for tightness in an area and mild discomfort right before the injury happens. The key to avoiding injury is programming short- and long-term plans, allowing you to predict when tension may be too high and backing off may be necessary. As well as listening to your body and adapting your plan when needed. Plans provide us with a starting point, something to build upon, but they are never set in stone.

Improvement Occurs During Recovery, Not Hard Efforts

Athletics have a way of inspiring us to go longer, faster, and harder because we can see our achievements before our eyes. Sports are one of those things in life that you become the result of your efforts. With that said, we can sometimes get carried away in our training and take it too far, too often. Don't get me wrong, pushing yourself is the only way to improve. You must introduce your body to a new challenging stimulus for it to adapt and improve. It is when you insert these hard efforts too often with too little break that trouble can start creeping up in the form of overtraining. Overtraining is the result of too much stimulus with too little time to adapt causing a decrease in performance. The key is noticing the signs of overtraining and cutting back your training before it becomes too late, and your performance deteriorates. Some common signs and symptoms to look out for overtraining are fatigue, increased resting heart rate, decrease or disrupted sleep, decrease in strength, irritability, decrease in muscle mass, depression, and joint pain.

If you are experiencing some of the descriptions above, then you may be overtraining. If so, here are some ideas you can employ to remedy the problem:

1. *Decrease activity:* Decrease your training by lowering your volume, frequency, and/or intensity for one to two weeks. If this doesn't work, then you may need to take time off completely.
2. *Participate in cross-training:* Cross-training reduces signs and symptoms of overtraining by reducing the stress muscles and joints commonly encountered during your typical training sessions.
3. *Relax your diet:* Relaxing your diet for a few days if it is typically very strict can help relieve overtraining. Conversely, eat healthier if you normally eat foods with poor nutritional value.
4. *Examine your diet:* Re-examine your diet, and make sure it is structured to your needs. Dietary needs change all the time and every athlete is unique. Knowing this, a typical athlete's diet should be composed of 55–60 percent carbohydrates, 30 percent fat (10 percent or less of which is from saturated fat), and 10–15 percent protein.
5. *Switch up your routine completely:* Upon returning to the gym after your break, engage in a routine with less structure for a while before training at your previous intensity.

When in Doubt, Listen to Your Body, Not a Book

What and When to Eat

Nutrition is a science pertaining to the relationship between food and its interactions with an organism including maintenance, growth, reproduction, health, and disease (The National Agricultural Library 1998). Food's relationship with athletes circles around athletes' diet and their bodies' response to that diet. Diet is the overall lifestyle habits concerned with eating food. Diets vary depending on the demands on an athlete's training schedule, competition, sleep, stress, age, and gender. Although food an athlete ingest maintains the same chemical composition regardless of who is consuming it, sufficient research has shown the athlete's metabolism, endocrine response, and utilization of that food will vary with the demands placed on the athlete's body, age, and gender (Feinman and Fine 2004; Noakes et al. 2005; Lockwood et al. 2008; Luscombe-Marsh et al. 2005; Symons et al. 2007).

Different Types of Carbohydrates: There are two main types of carbohydrates (carbs). Complex carbs and simple sugars. Complex carbs are what people consider your "healthy carbs." They take more time to enter your bloodstream and get to work, keeping your energy levels even and keeping your stomach full. Common examples of complex carb foods are whole grain and whole wheat, brown or wild rice, oatmeal, and beans. These are the foods you should be eating in the days leading up to a competition. Simple sugars on the other hand enter your bloodstream and spike up your energy levels quickly. These are good for right before and during a competition. Examples are sports drinks, juices, white bread, and many fruits (please see the chart on the following page).

Protein, the Foundation of Muscle: Proteins are used to build every structure in your body. Different amino acids (Amino acids are like puzzle pieces connecting to create different proteins) match up to build and reconstruct different proteins, which are used to make all the different components of your body. The same goes for muscles. Since your muscles need certain types of protein, they need certain types of amino acids to construct those proteins. This is why it is important to get protein from a variety of different sources; the best being animal sources because meat on animals is muscle, and you cannot get more biologically similar to muscle than muscle, and the other source is eggs. However, mixing plant-based protein sources can give you the right amino-acid pool as well. Also, when it comes to protein timing, Whey protein should be consumed around physical activity and casein protein before bed. Whey protein acts quicker, delivering much needed BCAAs to your muscles, while casein protein works over a longer period, keeping your body anabolic while you sleep. More on protein can be read in the next chapter.

Fat, an Endless Energy Supply: Fats are our primary fuel source, and the taboo of fat as unhealthy has finally lifted. However, we always have enough fat as fuel, which is why I focus on becoming a fat efficient athlete. Recent dietary recommendations lifted the upper limit of fat intake, focusing our awareness towards reducing saturated fat and trans fat while aiming for unsaturated and especially polyunsaturated fat. We have also learned it is not dietary cholesterol that leads to heart disease but excessive consumption of saturated and trans fats. The big take away here is keep saturated fat levels below 10% of dietary consumption and aim for polyunsaturated fats.

Complex Carbohydrates	Complex Carbohydrates (Cont.)	Simple Carbohydrates
• Apples • Apricots, dried • Artichokes • Asparagus • Brown rice • Buckwheat • Buckwheat bread • Cabbage • Carrots • Celery • Grapefruit • Lettuce • Muesli • Multigrain bread • Oat-bran cereal • Oatmeal • Okra • Oranges • Pears • Plums • Prunes • Spinach • Strawberries • Turnip greens • Whole barley • Wild rice • Yams • Zucchini	• Broccoli • Brussels sprouts • Cauliflower • Cucumbers • Dill pickles • Eggplant • Garbanzo beans • Kidney beans • Lentils • Lentils • Navy beans • Onions • Pinto beans • Potatoes • Radishes • Skim milk • Soy milk • Soybeans • Split peas • Yogurt, low fat	• All baked goods made with white flour • Bread made with white flour • Cake • Candy • Candy • Corn syrup • Fruit juice • Pasta made with white flour • Soda • Table sugar

Before Competition or Practice: When it comes to fueling up before a competition, athletes should focus mostly on carbohydrates with a little protein so it is ready to get to work once physical activity ceases. Carbs are your body's best energy source. Metabolizing quicker than fats and lasting longer than creatine. No matter what sport or position you play, whether it is explosive or endurance, your body needs carbs to fuel your muscles. Your diet should be composed of 55-60 percent carbs. Protein synthesis kicks in with as little as 4g of protein, so if I can sneak 4g of protein into my pre-workout snack it will speed up my post-workout recovery. The food you consume before practice or competition is as important as the food you consume after, since it takes 60-90 minutes for food to digest and enter the bloodstream.

After the Competition or Practice: After you're done, it is vital you consume a 3-4:1 carb-to-protein ratio immediately. The sooner you do this, the better the benefits. You have a two-hour window to get in these calories and maximize recovery, but ideally you want to do it within the first thirty minutes. The reason being, you just finished tearing apart and depleting your muscles, and now they must rebuild and refuel. With that said, if you cannot eat within two hours post activity, still consume something. It's better to be late than never. Muscles cannot rebuild if you do not give them the "tools" to rebuild (protein) and fuel to reenergize (carbs and fats). It is best if your carbs are a mix of complex carbs and simple sugars and your proteins have a high biological value (BV). A high BV means the protein most highly resembles what your body needs. Far too often we focus on protein after a workout to rebuild, but we must also focus on refueling as well as consuming anabolic foods such as dark leafy greens. These foods contain vitamins and minerals such as zinc, boron, magnesium, and vitamins A, B6, and C we need to stay anabolic.

Food Protein Rating—
Biological Value (BV)
1. Eggs (whole)—100
2. Eggs (whites)—88
3. Chicken/Turkey—79
4. Fish—70
5. Lean beef—69
6. Cow's milk—60
7. Unpolished rice—59
8. Brown rice—57
9. White rice—56
10. Peanuts—55
11. Peas—55
12. Whole wheat—49
13. Soy beans—47
14. Whole-grain wheat—44
15. Peanuts—43
16. Corn—36
17. Dry beans—34
18. White potato—34

Protein Supplement Protein Rating
1. Whey Protein Isolate—159
2. Whey Protein Concentrate—104
3. Casein—77
4. Soy—74

Chickpeas Are a Great Source of Boron and Coffee is an Excellent Source of Magnesium

All Hail Protein

Out of all the diets, athletes participate in during their attempts to get faster, get stronger, and go farther, perhaps the most engrossing and popular diet trends involve protein. In athletics protein is held to an almost sacred standard for skeletal-muscle tissue repair after training. The following chapter evaluates a variety of metabolic responses athletes undergo when consuming protein under a range of variables to determine what is the most effective amount of protein, when is the most appropriate protein timing, varying protein consumption protocols, and what are the detrimental effects of high-protein diets.

How much protein?

The first study by Campbell, Kreider, Ziegenfuss, La Bounty, Roberts, Burke, Landis, Lopez, and Antonio (2007) list the seven points of the International Society of Sports Nutrition's position on protein and exercise. The seven points relate to the intake of protein for healthy exercising individuals and are as follows:

1. Vast research supports the contention that individuals engaged in regular exercise training require more dietary protein than sedentary individuals.
2. Protein intakes of 1.4–2.0 g/kg/day for physically active individuals is not only safe but may improve the training adaptations to exercise training.
3. When part of a balanced, nutrient-dense diet, protein intake at this level is not detrimental to kidney function or bone metabolism in healthy, active persons.
4. While it is possible for physically active individuals to obtain their daily protein requirements through a varied, regular diet, supplemental protein in various forms is a practical way of ensuring adequate and quality protein intake for athletes.
5. Different types and quality of protein can influence amino-acid bioavailability following protein supplementation. The superiority of one protein type over another in terms of optimizing recovery and/or training adaptations remains to be convincingly demonstrated.
6. Appropriately timed protein intake is an important component of an overall exercise-training program, essential for proper recovery, immune function, and the growth and maintenance of lean body mass.
7. Under certain circumstances, specific amino-acid supplements, such as branched-chain amino acids (BCAAs), may improve exercise performance and recovery from exercise.

These basic recommendations set in place by the International Society of Sports Nutrition give registered dietitians, nutritionist, coaches, and athletes fundamental suggestions to follow.

Protein timing

Additional research from the International Society of Sports Nutrition by Kerksick, Harvey, Stout, Campbell, Wilborn, Kreider, Kalman, Ziegenfuss, Lopez, Landis, Ivy, and Antonio (2008) scrutinizes nutrient-timing protocols, determining the most effective methods for intake of carbohydrates, proteins, and fats regarding healthy exercising individuals. The International Society of Sports Nutrition summarized their findings into the following eight principles:

1. Maximal endogenous glycogen stores are best promoted by following a high-glycemic, high-carbohydrate (CHO) diet (600–1,000 g CHO or ~8–10 g CHO/kg/d), and ingestion of free amino acids and protein (PRO) alone or in

combination with carbohydrates before resistance exercise can maximally stimulate protein synthesis.

2. During exercise, carbohydrates should be consumed at a rate of thirty to sixty grams of CHO/hour in a 6–8 percent carbohydrate solution (eight to sixteen fluid ounces) every ten to fifteen minutes. Adding protein to create a CHO:PRO ratio of 3–4:1 may increase endurance performance and maximally promotes glycogen resynthesis during acute and subsequent bouts of endurance exercise.

3. Ingesting carbohydrates alone or in combination with protein during resistance exercise increases muscle glycogen, offsets muscle damage, and facilitates greater training adaptations after either acute or prolonged periods of supplementation with resistance training.

4. Post-exercise (within thirty minutes) consumption of carbohydrates at high dosages (8–10 g CHO/kg/day) have been shown to stimulate muscle glycogen resynthesis, while adding protein (0.2 g–0.5 g PRO/kg/day) to carbohydrates at a ratio of 3–4:1 (CHO: PRO) may further enhance glycogen resynthesis.

5. Post-exercise ingestion (immediately to three hours post) of amino acids, primarily essential amino acids, has been shown to stimulate robust increases in muscle protein synthesis, while the addition of carbohydrates may stimulate even greater levels of protein synthesis. Additionally, pre-exercise consumption of a carbohydrate and protein supplement may result in peak levels of protein synthesis.

6. During consistent, prolonged resistance training, post-exercise consumption of varying doses of carbohydrate and protein supplements in varying dosages have shown to stimulate improvements in strength and body composition when compared to control or placebo conditions.

7. The addition of creatine (Cr) (0.1 g Cr/kg/day) to a carbohydrate and protein supplement may facilitate even greater adaptations to resistance training.

8. Nutrient timing incorporates the use of methodical planning and eating of whole foods, nutrients extracted from food, and other sources. The timing of the energy intake and the ratio of certain ingested macronutrients are likely the attributes, which allow for enhanced recovery and tissue repair following high-volume exercise, augmented muscle protein synthesis, and improved mood states when compared with unplanned or traditional strategies of nutrient intake. Providing evidence that a combination of protein and carbohydrates prior, during, and after exercise will provide the best results in performance and recovery. These findings are applicable to every athlete's training regimen seeing that all athletes must take full advantage of their diet including effective timing if they want to attain the most gains possible.

Protein consumption

Hoffman, Ratamess, Kang, Falve, and Faigenbaum (2006) investigate the effect of protein intake on strength, body composition, and endocrine change in strength/power athletes. Participants were twenty-three experienced collegiate strength/power athletes participating in a twelve-week resistance training program comparing varying consumptions of protein; below recommended levels (BL; 1.0–1.4 g.kg-1.day-1; n = 8), recommended levels (RL; 1.6–1.8 g.kg-1.day-1; n = 7), and above recommended levels (AL; > 2.0 g.kg-1.day-1; n = 8). Participants were then assessed for strength (one-repetition maximum [1RM] bench press and squat) and body composition. Procedures include analyzing resting blood samples for total testosterone, cortisol, growth hormone, and insulin-like growth factor. Findings showed no differences in energy intake (3,171 +/− 577 kcal) between the groups. Moreover, energy intake for all groups was also below the recommended levels for strength/power athletes.

Results of the study showed no significant changes in body mass, lean body mass, or fat mass in any group. Significant improvements in 1RM bench press and 1RM squat were seen in all three groups; however, no differences between the groups were observed. Subjects in the above recommended levels group experienced a 22 percent and 42 percent greater change in 1RM squat and 1RM bench press than subjects in the recommended levels group; however, these differences were not significant. No significant changes were seen in any of the resting hormonal concentrations.

These findings suggest ingesting protein beyond recommended levels in collegiate strength/power athletes for body-composition improvements or alterations in resting hormonal concentrations will not show any further improvements than taking recommended dosage. With all the high-protein supplements on the market, these findings suggest the benefits of ingesting protein beyond recommended levels may be minimal at best, and athletes may have better results investing their resources in other safe supplementation methods and stacking (combining) protein with creatine or carbohydrates. It is also known that when too great a focus is placed on protein, athletes may miss out on other free-testosterone promoting nutrients such as boron and magnesium. For this reason, excessive protein should not be consumed, but rather a well-balanced diet with adequate protein intake is suggested for muscle growth.

Keep Whey Protein Consumption Under 20g/Serving and Casein Under 40g/Serving

A study by Roy (2008) investigates the new growing interest in bovine milk to see if there is justification in its growing popularity as a sports drink substitute, especially as a recovery agent after exercise. Roy examined the limited research and concluded that milk appears to be an effective post-resistance exercise beverage resulting in desirable acute alterations increasing muscle protein synthesis, leading to an improved net muscle-protein balance. What's more, when post-exercise milk consumption is combined with resistance training (twelve weeks minimum), greater increases in muscle hypertrophy and lean mass have been observed. Although research with milk is limited, there is some evidence to suggest that milk may be an effective post-exercise beverage for activities.

Additionally, low-fat milk has been shown to be as effective, if not more effective, than commercially available sports drinks as a rehydration beverage. For athletes in need of a more nutrient-dense beverage choice, milk represents a great alternative for those who partake in strength and endurance activities, compared to traditional sports drinks. Bovine low-fat fluid milk is a safe and effective post-exercise beverage for most individuals, except for those who are lactose intolerant. Roy notes further research is needed to better set forth the possible applications and efficacy of bovine milk in the field of sports nutrition. Roy's research is an appropriate example of how everyday foods and beverages can give athletes the same if not better results than sports supplements developed in labs and engineered by scientist. These results provide proof that natural foods should be the foundation of a healthy diet and supplements should be just that, supplementing a natural diet.

Supplementing Roy's work on milk as a sports drink substitute is research by Martinez-Lagunals, Ding, Bernard, Wang, and Ivy (2010) examining added protein's efficacy of a low-carbohydrate sports drink. Martinez-Languals and colleagues investigate the aerobic capacity characteristics of an isocaloric carbohydrate (CHO) plus protein (PRO) drink and a low-calorie carbohydrate plus protein drink against a traditional 6 percent carbohydrate sports beverage.

Milk is Shown to be Beneficial for Muscle Growth

Participants include twelve male and female trained cyclists who exercised on four separate occasions at intensities varying between 55 and 75 percent VO_2max for 2.5 hours and then at 80 percent VO_2max until fatigued. Supplements (255.4 +/– 9.1 mL) were provided every twenty minutes and consisted of a 4.5 percent carbohydrate plus 1.15 percent protein complex (CHO/PRO H), a 3 percent carbohydrate plus 0.75 percent protein complex (CHO/PRO L), a 6 percent carbohydrate supplement (CHO), or a placebo (PLA).

Results showed time to fatigue at 80 percent VO_2max was significantly longer ($p < 0.05$) during the carbohydrate (26.9 +/– 6.1 minutes, mean +/– SE), the CHO/PRO H (30.5 +/– 5.9 minutes), and the CHO/PRO L (28.9 +/– 6.5 minutes) trials compared with the placebo trial (14.7 +/– 3.4 minutes), with no significant differences among the CHO, CHO/PRO H, and CHO/PRO L treatments. Additionally, blood glucose, plasma insulin, and carbohydrate oxidation were elevated above placebo during the CHO, CHO/PRO H, and CHO/PRO L trials, whereas plasma-free fatty acids, rating of perceived exertion, and fat-oxidation values were lower during the CHO, CHO/PRO H, and CHO/PRO L trials compared with the placebo trial. Insignificant differences were observed in blood parameters occurred among the CHO, CHO/PRO H, and CHO/PRO L treatments.

I know that was a lot of acronyms, but basically these findings suggest adding protein to a carbohydrate-based sports drink will not improve endurance performance; however, because the addition of protein does not negatively impact efficacy, it can be recommended to add protein to low-carbohydrate sports beverages to enhance aerobic capacity and anabolism while limiting caloric intake and carbohydrate consumption. Combining the results of Martinez-Lagunals and colleagues' findings with Roy's (2008) findings, it appears low-fat chocolate milk because of its low-fat composition with a 3–4:1 carbohydrate-to-protein ratio is an excellent alternative to sports drinks.

Recovery Drinks with a 3-4:1 Carb-to-Protein Ratio Are Best for a Quick Recovery

While many sports focus on getting athletes as big and strong as possible, an equally large number of sports are hard pressed toward maintaining a low body-fat percentage and high strength-to-weight ratio. With respect to diets and weight loss, there is a decades old debate regarding which macronutrient restricted diet will promote the most weight loss. Recent research by Noakes, Keogh, Fosters, and Clifton (2005) shows that when on an energy-restricted diet high in protein and low in fat, the nutritional and metabolic benefits are equal and sometimes greater than those observed with a high carbohydrate diet.

Additional findings to support a high-protein diet were uncovered by Lockwood, Moon, Tobkin, Walter, Smith, Dalbo, Cramer, and Stout (2008) shows that when on a non-calorie-restricted diet consisting of high-protein, low-fat, and low-carbohydrate, overall nutrition intake improved, physiological adaptions to exercise increased, and muscle mass and time-to-exhaustion enhanced. Moreover, it was shown by Ivy, Res, Sprague, and Widzer (2003) that protein and carbohydrate supplementation increased endurance in athletes more than carbohydrate supplementation alone. However, the reason for the finding is unknown. With that said, athlete's desiring to reduce body fat in a safe manner while maintaining lean mass should use a high-protein, low-fat, and low-carbohydrate diet. Keeping in mind, excessive protein intake can also hinder progress and should, therefore, be consumed within recommended ranges.

With all this research revealing high-protein diets as an effective diet model for athletes looking to gain or maintain lean mass while increasing performance, the question, "why is protein so metabolically effective at building athletes?" comes to mind. Answers to why high-protein diets are effective at reducing body fat while maintaining lean mass in a safe manner may reside in a study titled "A Calorie Is a Calorie," by Feinman and Fine (2004). Feinman and Fine state the manner people view calories as all being created equal with respect to usable energy violates the second law of thermodynamics. It was pointed out that a calorie is not a calorie as far as the three macronutrients providing equal amounts of energy per calorie is concerned.

Researchers pointed out the second law of thermodynamics, something is lost and, therefore, balance is not to be expected, does not account for living things. The thermic effects of food (energy being used to breakdown the macronutrients into usable energy) is not equal. Fat uses 2–3 percent, carbohydrates 6–8 percent, and proteins 25–30 percent of their energy in the process of becoming usable energy for the body. Therefore, protein's high energy demands to be metabolized by the body naturally make it a less caloric energy substrate because of its own chemical makeup. This is partially due to protein containing nitrogen, which makes it harder to metabolize. The nitrogen in protein is also why high-protein dieters lose more initial weight than high-fat dieters, the nitrogen uses more water to metabolize and thus high-protein dieters can attribute most of their initial weight loss to water loss.

Proteins Use 25-30 Percent of Their Energy Becoming Usable Energy

On the other side of the coin, despite all the research supporting high-protein diets, Luscombe-Marsh, Noakes, Wittert, Keogh, Foster, and Clifton (2005) has shown slightly different results. Revealing in addition to high-protein diets promoting weight loss, high-fat diets have been shown equally effective at promoting fat loss and improving blood lipids. It is my opinion that this is a result of higher free-testosterone from a wider range of nutrient intake when focusing on high-fat diets.

Lemon (1991) gives a review of protein needs of strength athletes. Lemon highlights evidence indicating that actual protein requirements of strength athletes are higher than those of more sedentary individuals. Data also suggests the combination of high-protein/amino-acid diets combined with heavy resistance exercise training can enhance the development of muscle mass and strength. It is also of note novices may have higher needs than experienced strength athletes, and substantial individual variability exists. Furthermore, Norton and Layman (2006) showed the branched-chain amino acid leucine is necessary for protein synthesis in skeletal muscle after exercise. These findings suggest that, although inconclusive, high-protein/amino-acid diets specifically containing leucine among strength athletes may be beneficial in producing lean mass and strength.

Leucine Aids in Building Lean Muscle Mass and Strength

With all the research showing high-protein diets as an effective diet for athletes, it is important to point out chicken eggs, which are a standard in many high-protein diets were shown to be safe with respects to heart disease. Research conducted by Donald J. McNamara (2000) showed when an egg is consumed, it introduces a 100 mg change in dietary cholesterol and a 2.2 mg/dL change in plasma total cholesterol. Although these changes may seem significant, it is not the change in plasma total cholesterol that increases risk of heart disease but the ratio of low density lipoproteins (LDL) to high density lipoproteins (HDL), LDL:HDL, indicating heart disease. Furthermore, consuming an egg produces minimal changes in the LDL:HDL ratio, thus consuming an egg does not increase the risk of heart disease.

Eating Eggs Does Not Lead to Heart Disease

Additionally, it was discovered by Symons, Schutzler, Cocke, Chinkes, Wolfe, and Paddon-Jones (2007) in their research on the effects of aging on the body's anabolic response to a protein-rich meal; although differences in the concentration of amino acids in the plasma-precursor pool where noticed, aging does not impair muscle protein synthesis after eating a protein-rich food.

Aging Does Not Diminish Muscle Protein Synthesis

Potential detrimental effects

With a vast pool of research supporting high-protein diets, it is worth time examining potential damaging effects on the body by consuming a high-protein diet for a long term. Poortmans and Dellalieux (2000) investigated body builders and other well-trained athletes with high- and medium-protein intake, respectively, to shed light on excess protein and amino-acid intake and kidney function, leading to progressive kidney impairment. Participants underwent a seven-day nutrition record analysis as well as blood sample and urine collection to determine the potential renal consequences of high-protein intake. The data revealed that despite higher plasma concentration of uric acid and calcium, the group of body builders had renal clearances of creatinine, urea, and albumin that were within the normal range. The nitrogen balance for both groups became positive when daily protein intake exceeded 1.26 g/kg, but there were no correlations between protein intake and creatinine clearance, albumin excretion rate, and calcium excretion rate. Findings suggest that protein intake under 2.8 g/kg does not impair renal function in well-trained athletes as indicated by blood sample and urine collection.

Periods of Protein Intake Up To 2.8g/kg are Safe for Healthy Individuals

Martin, Armstrong, and Rodriquez (2005) also provide a review on increased dietary protein intake as a health concern in terms of the potential to initiate or promote renal disease. Martin and colleagues conclude, while protein restriction may be appropriate for treatment of existing kidney disease, there is no significant evidence for a detrimental effect of high-protein intake on kidney function in healthy persons after centuries of a high-protein Western diet. With that said, healthy athletes may continue to consume high-protein diets unless their body's renal function tells them otherwise, in which they should seek medical attention.

In closing, moderate to high levels of protein appear to be an essential and healthy component in an athlete's diet. Supplementing protein with carbohydrates, creatine, and branched-chain amino acids increases the anabolic effects of protein further than protein ingestion alone. Although protein is an effective agent for physiological change in athlete composition and performance, it is worthy of note that a proper training regimen must but utilized with proper nutrition to trigger the endocrine responses and physiological changes possible through proper sports nutrition. Further reading should be done regarding the body's response to protein under additional circumstances such as first thing upon waking up, prior to bed, protein's effect on concentration, and gender differences concerning protein consumption. As a popular macronutrient, extensive research has been done on protein that is beyond the scope of this book.

Stacking Protein with Other Safe Supplements Enhances Anabolic Effects

It seems everyone is looking for the ultimate supplement. The one that is going to make you the "perfect athlete," and they are willing to spend hundreds of dollars doing it. I am not saying supplements do not work, some have been proven to work tremendously. However, the best and safest supplement for athletic performance is everywhere, and, it is free. It's water!

Water itself is not generally thought of as a supplement, rather a necessity of life. Understanding this, a supplement by definition is something that completes or enhances something else. Think of water as an enhancing performance factor in the same way you think of caffeine, creatine monohydrate, or BCAAs. When viewed in this manner, most people will be more on top of their water consumption.

The human body during adulthood is made up of approximately 70 percent water (allaboutwater.org). That is a lot of water. With that said, roughly 75 percent of all Americans are suffering from dehydration. This lack of water in our system accounts for many problems in our everyday lives, such as overeating. Over one-third of Americans mistake the thirst mechanism for hunger, causing them to eat more than they need. This can be remedied by having one glass of water instead of a snack to curb your appetite. Furthermore, besides causing you to eat more, when you are even mildly dehydrated, your metabolism can slow down by up to 3 percent.

If you do not think those facts are enough to cause you to start drinking more water, listen to this. Being dehydrated is the main source of daytime fatigue; it can lead to short-term memory loss and even lack of focusing ability. So, next time you want to get up from your desk and grab a coffee, grab a tall glass of water instead.

Knowing how important water is for performance, I need to clear up an old myth that dehydration leads to performance decline. Athletes become dehydrated during peak performance all the time as a natural part of the activity without any issues. Since athletes sweat during physical activity, their electrolyte balance stays in check with their fluid loss. It is pre-performance dehydration that leads to dilemmas during competition, because now the sodium-potassium pump is not balanced and performance will readily decline.

Hydrating Prior to Competition is Essential for Avoiding Performance Decline

It's as obvious as the value of leg day, drinking enough water is very important for your body. Moreover, it is readily available and for a good price. Make sure you drink roughly ten glasses of water a day (depending on your size) and notice your workouts and everyday activities soar!

I'm going to lay it right out there. The more fat you have, the fatter you will get. Do not take that statement the wrong way. Current dietary recommendations have lifted the upper limit of total fat, science has revealed it is excessive levels of saturated and trans fat that lead to heart disease. But this lesson is focused on lipid (fat) accumulation or fat stored in the body.

The human body is designed to be as efficient as possible. It's a trait leftover from when we had to worry about when we were going to get our next meal. Our body didn't want to waste any precious energy, so it became a master of efficiency.

Because of this, our body likes fat and not muscle. This is because muscle is three times more metabolically active (uses more energy) than fat. For our body to sustain a pound of fat, it takes two calories per day, but to sustain a pound of muscle, it takes six.

This is why when we stop resistance training, our muscles shrink. Our body does not want the extra work of sustaining muscle. If it's not necessary, it ditches the extra weight.

Fat also "knows" muscle is a waste of energy. Visceral fat located beneath your abdomen muscles releases substances that lessen the quality and volume of muscle. This reduction in muscle mass slows down your body's metabolism, which in turn leads to even more fat gain.

The More Fat Cells You Have, The Easier it is to Build Additional Fat Stores

On top of that, visceral fat messes with hormones that balance metabolism. Slowing down those hormones so there is less calorie burn and more fat accumulation.

Don't worry. There is a way to fight back! Build more muscle. The more muscle you have, the more metabolically active your body is, and the more fat will be burned. Just how fat leads to more fat, less fat leads to less fat.

Epilogue

Upon finishing this book, I hope you have gained a basic understanding of the concepts of sport and exercise science as well as an interest in the field. I decided to keep the chapters short because there are so many different philosophies and I believe there is something to learn from all of them. In my personal experience, I have read endless research contradicting other research as well as acquired multiple certifications in sport, fitness, and health. All of which preach something slightly different. By keeping my book short, it gives you more time to explore other ideas. As I state in the title, "athletes in search of excellence," excellence cannot be achieved by only examining one mentor's viewpoint.

All I ask is upon reading this book, you have a direction to guide your athletic career. Please take the knowledge and years of experience collected and devise a plan towards your goals. Use PROformance Training Systems to develop your (or your client's) programs, because a clear path is the only path to excellence.

Your Journey Towards Excellence Should Encompass A Range of Perspectives

Appendix A: Charts and Diagrams
PROformance Training Systems Theme Breakdown

Mechanical	Learn	Prepare	Fortify	Potential
	Mobility *Sets* 2-3 *Reps* 12-15 *Rest* 60 s *Intensity* 1%-40%	Functional Stability *Sets* 3 *Reps* 12-15 *Rest* 30-45 s *Intensity* 50%-75%	Muscular Endurance *Sets* 3 *Reps* 12-15 *Rest* < 30 s *Intensity* 50%-75%	Max Power *Sets* 3-6 *Reps* 1-10 *Rest* 3-5 min *Intensity* 45% Or 10% Body Weight
	Corrective *Sets* 2-3 *Reps* 12-15 *Rest* 60 s *Intensity* 40%-60%	Neuromuscular Efficiency *Sets* 3 *Reps* 12-15 *Rest* 30-45 s *Intensity* 50%-75%	Hypertrophy *Sets* 3-4 *Reps* 4-12 *Rest* 45 s-2.5 min *Intensity* 75%-85%	Advanced Movement Systems *Sets* 3-6 *Reps* 1-10 *Rest* 3-5 min *Intensity* 100%
			Heavy Power *Sets* 4-6 *Reps* 1-4 *Rest* 3-5 min *Intensity* 85%-100%	
Metabolic	Learn	Prepare	Fortify	Potential
	Metabolic Stimulation *HR* 50%-60% *Reps* = Vary *Rest* = As needed	Aerobic Elevation *HR* 60%-80% *Reps* 1 *Rest* = Steady State	Threshold Development *HR* 80%-92% *Rest* 5:1 Ratio	Specific Movements *As Appropriate*
			Aerobic Capacity *HR* 92%-100% *Rest* 2:1-1:1 Ratio	Specific Skills *As Appropriate*
			Anaerobic Expansion *HR* 95%-100% *Rest* 1:3-1:5 Ratio	
Energy Refuel	Muscle Fiber Activation			
50% = 20-30 s 75% = 40 s 85%-90% = 60 s 100% = 3 min	Type I *Activation* 0% *Peak* 60% *Max* 80%	Type IIa *Activation* 60% *Peak* 85% *Peak* 100%	Type IIb *Activation* 90% *Peak* 100%+ *Max* 100%+	*These variables are for common use and can be adjusted.

The Proper Sequence of
Athletic Progression

Functional Movement

Mechanical Integrity

Metabolic Capacity

Specific Skills

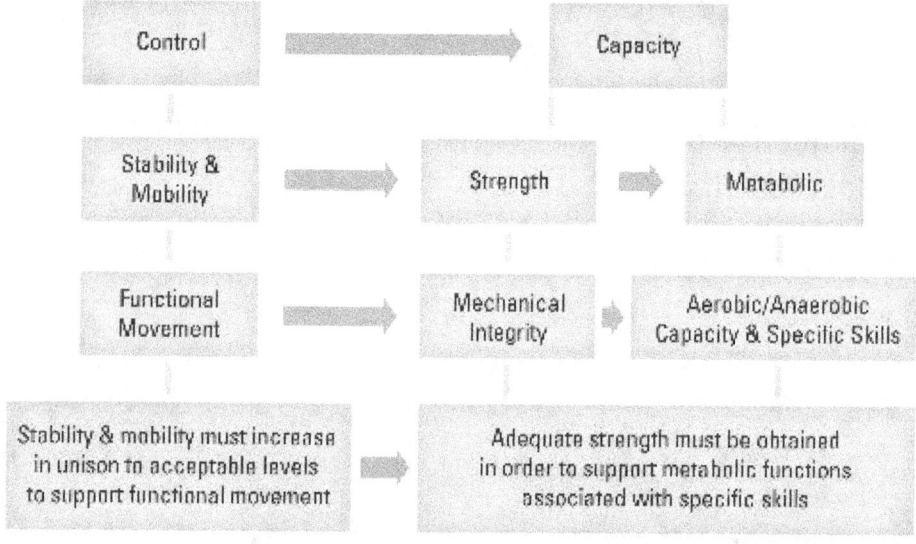

Survival

Avoid Pain &
the Unfamiliar

Improper
Movement
Patterns

Muscle
Imbalances

Poor
Arthrokinematics

Injury

Humans by nature are creatures of extreme efficiency. As a result we take the path of least resistance. If we are weak in certain areas, improper movement patterns can occur. This leads to muscle imbalances and poor arthro-kinematics (joint movement) that leads to injury. Our natural survival instincts tell us to avoid movements that cause pain or are unfamiliar even if they are natural. This leads to further pain and injury, creating an ongoing cycle.

We must re-educate our body to perform these basic movement patterns correctly in order to reduce injury and maximize performance. By relearning proper biomechanics from the beginning, we are allowing our bodies to perform in harmony with itself.

PROformance Training Systems

Functional Integrated Movements	Mechanical	Theme	Metabolic	Constant Evaluation & Systems Adaption
	Advanced Movement Systems & Max Power	Potential	**Specific Skills & Movements**	
	Maximize mechanical performance to allow optimal specific skills capability		Master movements and reactions to the demands of sport	
	Muscular Development III *Heavy Power*	Fortify	**Anaerobic Expansion**	
	Maximize connective tissue excitability and efficiency		Expand upon anaerobic capacity by implementing high intensity repetitions	
	Muscular Development II *Hypertrophy*		**Aerobic Capacity**	
	A hybrid between muscular development I & III		Improve the capacity at which oxygen can get to working muscles	
	Muscular Development I *Muscular Endurance*		**Threshold Development**	
	Increase the performance of metabolic pathways associated with repetitive muscle contraction		Establish resistance to fatigue at the ventilatory/ lactic threshold	
	Functional Stability & Neuromuscular Efficiency	Prepare	**Aerobic Elevation**	
	Improve motor control		Introduce aerobic elevation strategies to raise ventilatory threshold, increasing aerobic capacity	
	Basic Mobility & Corrective Strategies	Learn	**Metabolic Stimulation**	
	Work on any muscle imbalances & joint dysfunctions		Elevate heart rate in a novice & non-sports specific manner	

Mental Foundation & Support Structure
Motivation | Dedication | Resources

The PROformance Training Systems Progression Model

	Mechanical	Theme	Metabolic	
Functional	Advanced Movement Systems *Power & Max Integrated Movement*	Potential	Anaerobic Expansion *VO$_2$ Max & Repetitions Maturity*	Constant
Integrated	Muscular Development *Endurance & Strength Enhancement*	Fortify	Threshold Capacity *Improve Work Capacity and Race Pace*	Evaluation &
	Neuromuscular Efficiency *Improve Fire Order & Rate Efficiency*	Prepare	Aerobic Elevation *Raise Anaerobic Threshold*	Systems
Movements	Basic Mobility & Functional Stability *Re-educate, Proprioception, Balance*	Learn	Metabolic Stimulation *Elevate Heart Rate*	Adaption

How Long Should Each Theme Last?

PROformance Training Systems Theme Duration Breakdown				
Phase	**Metabolic**	**Mechanical**	**Duration (Weeks)**	**Resistance Phase Breakdown**
Learn	Aerobic Pace	Corrective	8–16	1/3
		Stability		
	Long and Slow Distance	Endurance		
Prepare	Long Intervals	Hypertrophy	4–6	1/2
	Tempo and Race Pace	Strength		
Fortify	VO$_2$Max	Explosive Power	2–4	1
	Short Repetition			
Potential	Aerobic	Plyometrics/ Corrective	1–3	Varies

Muscle Fiber-Type Activation Thresholds

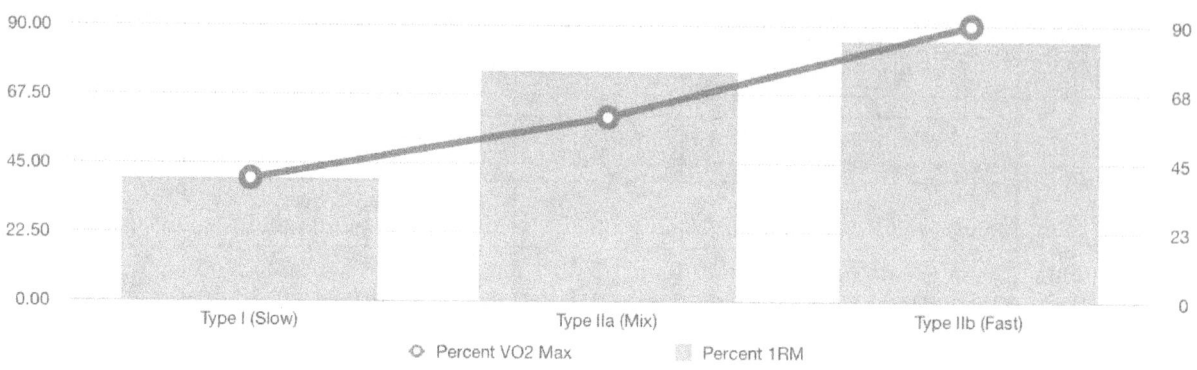

How Much Is Enough?

PROformance Training Systems Exercise Recommendation Chart					
Type of Activity		**Lose Ability**	**Maintain Ability**	**Gain Ability**	**Activity Duration**
Mechanical	Metabolic	Training Frequency (Days Per Week)			Minutes
Basic Mobility and Strength	Weight Control/ Maintenance	1–2	3	4–5	30
Hypertrophy (Muscle Size)	Competitive Endurance	<3	3–4	5–6	45–90
Athletic Strength	Competitive Conditioning (Nonendurance Athletes)	1–2	3	4–5	45–60
Competitive Power	Basic Cardiovascular Health	1	2	3–4	30–45

Mechanical Theme

Mob. > Corr. > Func. Stability > NM Efficiency > Muscular Endurance > Hypertrophy > Heavy Power > Max Power > AMS.

Metabolic Theme

Met. Stim. > Aero. Elevation > Thresh. Development > Aero. Capacity > An. Expansion > Spec. Movements > Spec. Skills

Date	Warm-Up		Cooldown		Primary Focus Movements
	Exercise	*Duration*	*Exercise*	*Duration*	Knee Hinge
__/__/__					Hip Hinge
					Vertical Push
					Vertical Pull
					Horizontal Push
					Horizontal Pull
					Core

Activity	Sets	Reps/Time	Weight/Distance	Rest

Mechanical Training Progression				
Method of Training	**Sets**	**Reps**	**Rest (s)**	**%1RM**
Corrective	2–3	12–15	60	40–60
Stabilization	3	12–15	30–45	50–70
Muscular Endurance	3	12–15	Up to 30	50–75
Hypertrophy/Strength	3–4	6–12	45–120	75–85
Heavy Power	5–6	1–5	180–300	85–100
Max Power	3–6	1–10	180–300	30–45 or 10% BW

Objective (Goal) of Training	Repetitions
Muscular Endurance	15–20+
Hypertrophy (Size)	8–12
Strength	4–8
Power	1–4(Heavy) or 6–10 (Fast & Light)

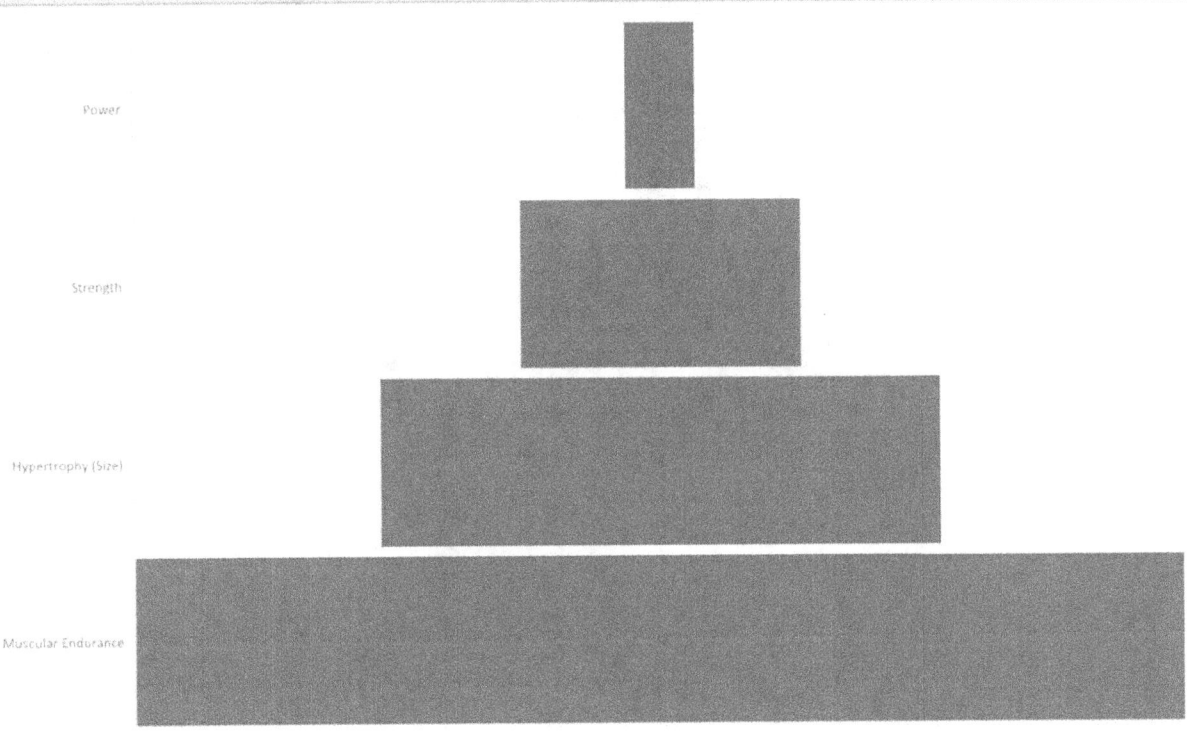

Rest Intervals by Time (Seconds)

Goal of Training	Time
Muscular Endurance	10–30 sec.
Hypertrophy (Size)	30–90 sec.
Strength	2–3 min. (120–180 sec.)
Power	3–5 min. (180–300 sec.)

Power

Strength

Hypertrophy (Size)

Muscular Endurance

Crossing the Lactic Threshold

1

Aerobic = Pyruvate

2

Go Anaerobic > Fermentation Occurs > Produces Lactate > Acidosis & Metabolites > Cause Fatigue & Discomfort

Crossing the Ventilitory Threshold

3

Body Attempts to Buffer Pyruvate
=
Buffering Produces CO_2 & Water

4

Exhale Harder to Rid the Body of CO_2 > Cross Over Ventilitory Threshold > Causes Heavier Breathing > Enventual Slow Down or Bonk Because You Cannot Get in Enough O_2

Work to Rest Intervals for Rep-Based Training

Repetitions	Rest
1-3	4-5 min
4-6	2-4 min
7-8	1 min
9-10	45-60 s
11-12	30-45 s
13-15+	< 30 s

Work to Rest Ratios for Time-Based Training

Activity	Ratio	Rest
5-10 s	1:6-1:12	1 min
15-30 s	1:3-1:4	1-1.5 min
1-3 min	1:1	1-3 min
3-5 min	1:1-2:1	1.5-5 min

Training Zones by Percent Max Heart Rate

	Training Zone	Heart Rate Range (%)
Aerobic	Warm up	50–60
	Recovery Pace	60–70
	Easy Runs & Long Runs	70–80
Anaerobic	Ventilatory Training/Lactic Threshold Pace	80–90
	VO_2max	92–98
	Repetition Pace	95–100

Hill Prescription

Length	Time	Intensity	Rest	Incline
Short	8-10 s	100%		12%-15%
Medium	20-30 s	95%-100%	60-180 s	8%-10%
Long	60-90 s	85%-95%		4%-6%

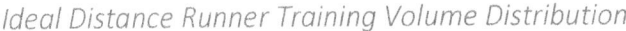

Type of Training	Percent of Training Volume	Percent of Max Heart Rate	Purpose of Activity
Aerobic	80%-90% (90% for base building)	65%-80%	Improve fat utilization.
Ventilatory Threshold	10%	80%-90%	Become more efficient at race pace.
VO$_2$max Intervals	7%	85%-95% (Potentially peaking at 98% for moments)	Increase VO$_2$max.
Sprint Repetitions	3%	95%+	Increase running efficiency and speed.

Ideal Distance Runner Training Volume Distribution

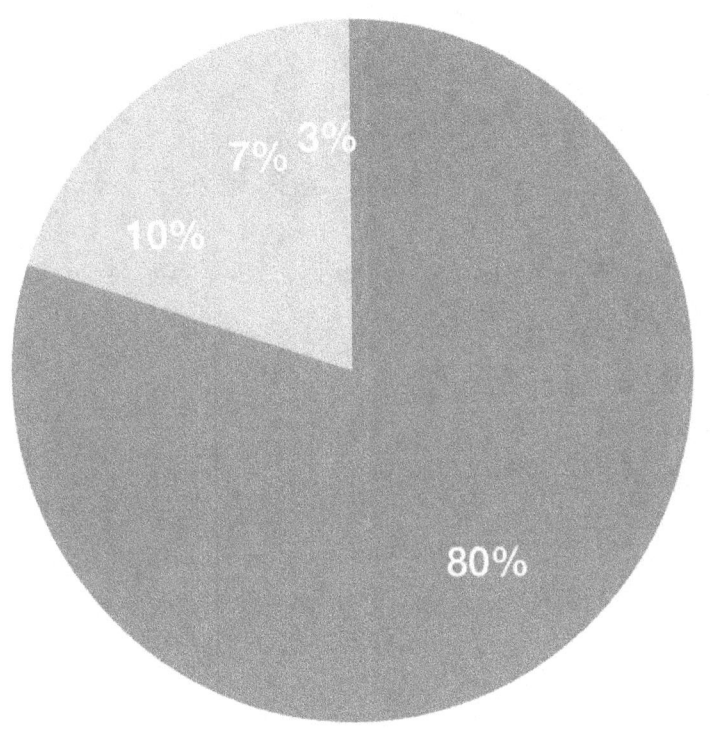

Aerobic
Race Pace
VO2 Max Intervals
Sprint Repetitions

Muscle Fiber Activation Thresholds by Heart Rate

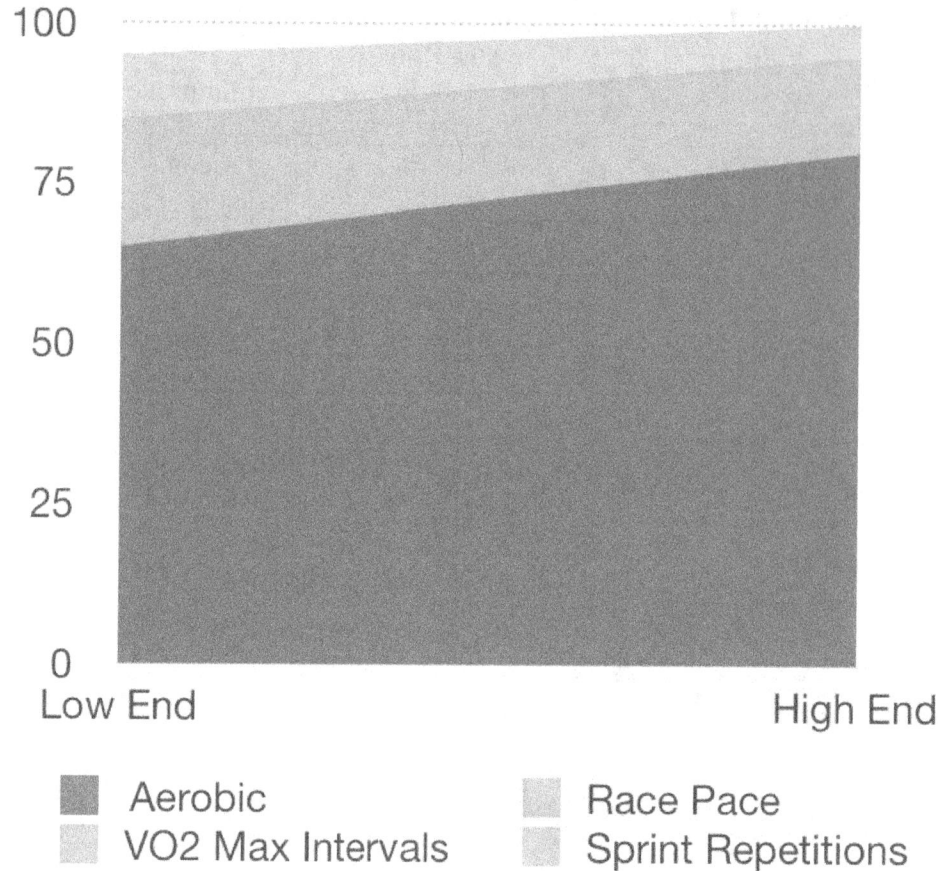

Sample Periodization Schedule

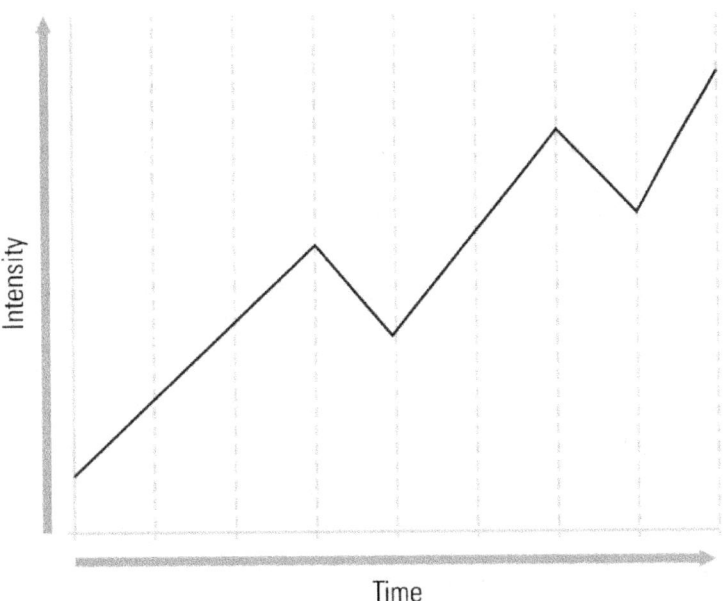

Thank You Coaches

Bold Lines Act as Cliff Notes

PROformance Training Systems Teaches You How to Organize Training Methods

Phosphagen & Glycolysis = Anaerobic; Aerobic = With Oxygen

Athletes Need to Progress in The Proper Sequence to Reach Their True Potential

Control Before Capacity

Stability and Mobility in Unison

Strength Comes Before Increasing Metabolic Ability

As We Age, We Take Movement Shortcuts That Lead to Injury

Social and Mental Support is as Valuable to Performance as Physical Conditioning

Mechanical Focuses on Strengthening Our Structure and Metabolic on Our Engine

Perform Mechanical Training Before Metabolic Training

Warm-Up for 10-20 Min Prior to Intense Physical Activity

Stretching and Pressure Relieve Tight Muscles

Perform a Dynamic Warm-Up Before Exercise and Static Stretching After Exercise

High BMI is Positively Correlated with All-Cause Mortality

Ergogenic Supplementation is Proven to Aid in Altering Body Composition

Quality of Life Decreases as Body Composition Increases to Unhealthy Levels

Body Composition Measurement Devices are Still Prone to Error

Ergogenic Aids Were Shown to Increase Lean Mass

Body Composition is an Accurate Indicator of Health Risk

Concurrent Training is More Effective Than Linear Training

In One Study, 2-3 Sets Was 46% Better for Strength Training Than a Single Set

Strength Training Does Not Hinder Endurance Athletes

Multiple Sets Deliver Compound Benefits

Exercise When Time Allows, Rather than Struggling for a Specific Time of Day

Recovery Time is Essential for Progress

Micro = Days; Meso = Weeks; Macro = Years

20 min very Strenuous/35 Min High Intensity = Muscle Growth, Sugar and Fat Metabolism

There is a Motivation Gene That is a Large Contributor to Excellence

Olympic Potential is More Common Than You May Think

GH Levels Increase with Compound Lower-body Strength Training

Adding Sleep Increases GH Levels, Potentially Offsetting the Effects of a Poor Diet

Five Sets of 75% 1RM Increases Anabolic Response During Bench Press

Three Sets at 75-80% 1RM Increases Anabolic Response During Leg Exercises

Multiple Bouts of Heavy-Resistance Training Increases Muscle Mass

Heavy-Resistance and High-Volume Training Increase Anabolic Hormones

Heavy-Long-Rest & Moderate-Short-Rest Produce Anabolic Responses

Training Above Lactate Threshold Increases Lean Mass & Fat Reduction

Free-Testosterone Levels Are Significant to Muscle Mass

Estrogen Enhances Endurance Performance

What Are You Doing Differently Today to Get You Beyond Yesterday?

It's A Combination of Hard Hard-Days and Easy Easy-Days That Lead to Adaption

Adaption is The Accord Between Repeated Exposure and Frequent Change

Systemic > Increased Active Musculature > More Required Blood Flow > Increased Heart Rate > Higher Energy Expenditure

Adequate Tension in Your Muscles Keeps Them Responsive

Reduce Speed Work, Plyometrics, and Power Training if You Become Lethargic

Strength is Increased with Heavy Sets of Five Reps or Less

Plyometrics Help You Cover More Distance with Each Step

"Launch Time" is the Amount of Time Your Foot is in Contact with the Ground

Your Ability to React Quickly is Essential in all Sports

Overtraining Will Diminish Reactive Strength

Keep Whey Protein Consumption Under 20g/Serving and Casein Under 40g/Serving

Milk is Shown to be Beneficial for Muscle Growth

Recovery Drinks with a 3-4:1 Carb-to-Protein Ratio Are Best for a Quick Recovery

Proteins Use 25-30 Percent of Their Energy Becoming Usable Energy

Leucine Aids in Building Lean Muscle Mass and Strength

Eating Eggs Does Not Lead to Heart Disease

Aging Does Not Diminish Muscle Protein Synthesis

Periods of Protein Intake Up To 2.8g/kg are Safe for Healthy Individuals

Stacking Protein with Other Safe Supplements Enhances Anabolic Effects

Chickpeas Are a Great Source of Boron and Coffee is an Excellent Source of Magnesium

Hydrating Prior to Competition is Essential for Avoiding Performance Decline

The More Fat Cells You Have, The Easier it is to Build Additional Fat Stores

Programs must Include Plyometric and Stabilization Exercises for Optimal Results

Vertical Jump Height is the Gold Standard of Measuring Power Output

Six Weeks of Plyometric Training Show an Improvement in Athletic Ability

Knee Injury Prevention Programs Should be Included Throughout Programing

Sprint Training is an Effective and Efficient Substitute for Plyometric Training

Plyometrics Increase Pure Applicable Power

Sprinting is a Harmony of Explosive Power and Delicate Proprioception

More Strength → More Force Production = More Speed with Reduced Energy Use = Faster Overall Pace with Less Effort

Plyometrics Improve Reciprocal Inhibition

Fascial Training Improves Power and Speed

Properly Executing Movement Patterns is Essential for Athletic Success

The Twelve Ounce Curl is NOT an Athletic Movement Pattern!

Multijoint-Multiplanar Exercises Improve Overall Mechanics

Phosphagen = <10 s; Glycolysis = 2 min; Oxidative = >2 min

Training in Unstable Positions Improves Stable Performance but Not Vice Versa

Don't Train Like a Sea Squirt

Deceleration Training Is Essential for Injury Prevention

HIIT is More Beneficial Than a Long Run for Ball Sports

Compound Exercises Increase Strength Quicker than Isolation Exercises

70% of Strength Gains Happen During the First Set

Heavy Breathing Upon Completing an Interval is Known as EPOC

HIIT is an Effective and Efficient Alternative to Traditional Exercise

Research Shows HIIT to be an Effective Substitute for Traditional Exercise

As Little as Two Weeks of Sprint Training Can Improve Endurance Capacity

Sprint Training Maintains Progress, While Saving Time

Sprinting Adaptions Vary Depending on Exercise Prescription

Walking is a Valuable Substitute for Athletes Who Cannot Run

Walking is Effective for Populations That Should Avoid High Stress Training

Athletes Should Use New Technologies to Monitor Their Health

Being Fit Reduces Mortality and Cancer Risk

With the Potential to Save 1 in 4 Lives, Learning How to Strength Train is Invaluable

We All Need More Health Education to Reduced Mortality

Increases in Cardiovascular Health are Related to Decreases in Healthcare Cost

Fitness and Health Care Professionals Need to Work Together

ACSM Recommends at Least 150 Minutes of Moderate-Intensity Exercise Per Week

Vitals Sharing is a Valuable Link Between Fitness and Medical Professionals

Medical and Health Professionals Should Have an Understanding of Fitness Training

Aerobic Conditioning Allows for Easier use of Fats as Fuel

A Higher Percentage of Fat is Used as Fuel During Lower Intensity Activity

High Intensity Exercise Relies Primarily on the Phosphagen and Glycolysis System

Percentage of Fat Metabolism is Higher in Exercising than Non-Exercising Muscles

Calorie Supplementation During Exercise Delays Our Use of Fat as Fuel

There Are Benefits to Exercise That Calorie Restriction Alone Does Not Provide

Reduced Rest Between Sets Utilizes More Fat as Fuel

All Races and Genders Metabolize Substrates Relatively the Same

During Exercise, Glucose Supplementation is Recommended Over Fat Consumption

Concurrently Using Two Training Modalities in a Single Session Alters Each Modalities

Catastrophe Theory Implies Fatigue is Induced Within Muscles

Central Governor Model Suggest Fatigue Keeps Us from Harming Ourselves

CNS Theories of Fatigue State the Limits of the Body Are Set by the Mind

Task Dependency Model States the CNS and PNS Work Synergistically

Task-Failure Model Suggest the Exercise Modality is Responsible for Fatigue

Psycholobiological Model States Motivation Keeps Fatigue at Bay

To Engage in Flow, Skill and Challenge Must be in Harmony

Success Follows Desire and Desire Stems from Past Success

Sports are a Perfect Domain for Sparking Creativity

Athletes as a Demographic Enjoy Exploring, Novelty, and Risk

Active Participation is More Productive than Passive Involvement

Classrooms can Learn from Videogames

Game-Based Mechanics Improve Attraction, Participation, and Retention in Sports

Carbohydrates Keep Fatigue at Bay Better Than BCAAs

Lactate Distributes Energy Throughout the Body

Lactate Clears More Easily During Aerobic Activity

Active Recovery Between Exercise Bouts Accelerates Lactate Clearance

Pyruvate Causes the Burning Sensation in Muscles

Ventilatory Threshold Training Improves Repetitive Sprint Ability

A Simple Talk Test Can Let You Know You Are Performing Anaerobically

Numerous Mechanisms Cause Fatigue

Rest Intervals Determine the Outcome of a Session as Much as Reps, Sets, and Weights

The Onset of Fatigue is Not Dependent on Joint Angle

Increasing the Contraction Speed of a Muscle Induces Fatigue Sooner

Long Runs Should be 20%-30% of Your Weekly Mileage

Race Pace Training is About Time Spent Training at Race Pace, Not Faster

The Higher the Intensity, the Less Time We Need Training at That Intensity

Fat is 12 Times More Efficient Than Carbohydrates

Your Race Pace is Determined from a Multitude of Variables

Evolution Made Us Efficient at Burning Fat, Training Improves That Gift

Most of an Endurance Athlete's Progress Occurs Below the Ventilatory Threshold

Positive Affirmation is Mind Over Matter

Positive Affirmation Will Help You in all Areas of Life

The Mind Cannot Tell the Difference Between Visualization Techniques and Reality

Make a Simple Plan and Execute

Reflexive Intelligence is What Allows Us to Perform Without Thinking

Our Best Sleep Generally Occurs from 11:00 PM – 7:00 AM

Lack of Sleep has a Similar Consequence as Overtraining

Muscles Have Better Access to Nutrients and Oxygen Than Ligaments and Tendons

Light Activity Speeds Recovery

Stretching and Pressure Point Therapy Relieves Muscle Cramps

We Need Periods of Reduced Intensity After High Intensity to Adapt and Improve

Weak Glutes & Core as Well as Tight Hip Flexors & Hamstrings Arise from Sitting

Tightness is a Sensation, Muscles May be Short & Contracted or Lengthened and Taut

Improvement Occurs During Recovery, Not Hard Efforts

Your Journey Towards Excellence Should Encompass A Range of Perspectives

When in Doubt, Listen to Your Body, Not a Book

Bibliography

ACSM issues new recommendations on quantity and quality of exercise. 2014, November. ASCM. http://acsm.org/about-acsm/media-room/news-releases/2011/08/01/acsm-issues-new-recommendations-on-quantity-and-quality-of-exercise. Accessed 16 November 2017.

Ahtiainen, J. P., A. Pakarinen, M. Alen, W. J. Kraemer, and K. Häkkinen. 2005. "Short Vs. Long Rest Period between the Sets in Hypertrophic Resistance Training: Influence on Muscle Strength, Size, and Hormonal Adaptions in Trained Men." *Journal of Strength and Conditioning Research* 19 (3): 572–82.

Allen, D. G., G. D. Lamb, and H. Westerblad. 2008. "Skeletal Muscle Fatigue: Cellular Mechanisms." *Physiological Reviews* 88 (4): 287–332. https://doi.org/10.1152/physrev.00015.2007. Accessed 16 November 2017.

Amann, M., S. M. Marcora, L. Nybo, T. A. Duhamel, T. D. Noakes, V. Jaquinandi, J. L. Saumet, P. Abraham, B. T. Ameredes, M. Burnley, A. M. Jones, S. C. Gandevia, J. E. Butler, and J. L. Taylor. 2008. "Viewpoint: Fatique Mechanisms Determining Exercise Performance: Integrative Physiology Is Systems Physiology." *Journal of Applied Physiology* 104 (5): 1543–44.

American Society of Exercise Physiologist. 2014. "What Is Exercise Physiology?" http://www.asep.org. Accessed 16 November 2017.

Andrew, D., J. Kovaleski, R. Heitman, and T. Robinson. 2010. "Effects of Three Modified Plyometric Depth Jumps and Periodized Weight Training on Lower Extremity Power." *Sport Journal* 13 (1): 4.

Ann Yancy, W. S Jr., M. K. Olsen, J. R. Guyton, R. P. Bakst, and E. C. Westman. 2004. "A Low- carbohydrate, Ketogenic Diet Vs. a Low-Fat Diet to Treat Obesity and Hyperlipidemia: A Randomized, Controlled Trial." *Annals of Internal Medicine* 140 (10): 769–77.

Aragon, A. A., and B. J. Schoenfeld. 2013. "Nutrient Timing Revisited: Is There a Post-exercise Anabolic Window?" *Journal of the International Society of Sports Nutrition* 10 (1): 5. https://doi.org/10.1186/1150-2783-10-5.

Baechle, T. R., and R. Earle. 2000. "Cardiovascular and Respiratory Anatomy and Physiology: Responses to Exercise." In *Essentials of Strength and Conditioning*, edited by G. G. Haff and N. T. Triplett, 115–36. Champaign, IL: Human Kinetics.

Ball, S. (2016). "A Strength Training Program for Your Home." *American College of Sports Medicine*, http://www.acsm.org/public-information/articles/2016/10/07/a-strength-training-program-for-your-home. Accessed 14 November 2017.

Barry, B., and R. Enoka. 2007. "The Neurobiology of Muscle Fatigue: 15 Years Later." Integrative and Comparative Biology 47 (4): 465–73. https://doi.org/10.1093/icb/icm047.

Bonen, A. 2000. "Lactate Transporters (MCT Proteins) in Heart and Skeletal Muscle." *Medicine and Science in Sports and Exercise* 32 (4): 778–89.

Bönig, D., and N. Maassen. 2008. "Point: Counterpoint: Lactic Acid Is/Is Not the Only Physicochemical Contributor to the Acidosis of Exercise." *Journal of Applied Physiology* 105:358–59.

Böning, D. G. Strobel, R. Beneke, and N. Maassen. 2005. "Lactic Acid Still Remains the Real Cause of Exercise-Induced Metabolic Acidosis." *Journal of Physiology-Regulatory, Integrative and Comparitive Physiology* 289 (3): 902–3.

Borkan, G. A., D. E. Hults, S. G. Gerzof, A. H. Robbins, and C. K. Silert. 1983. "Age Changes in Body Composition Revealed by Computer Tomography." *The Journal of Gerontol* 38 (6): 673–77.

Brooks, G. A. 2000. "Intra- and Extra- Cellular Lactate Shuttles." *Medicine & Science in Sports & Exercise* 32 (4): 790–99.

Bryant, C. X. 2014. "Fitness as Pharmacy." *IDEA Fitness Journal* 11 (9): 76–77.

Burgomaster, K. A., G. J. Heigenhauser, and M. J. Gibala. 2006. "Effect of Short-Term Sprint Interval Training on Human Skeletal Muscle Carbohydrate Metabolism During Exercise and Time-trial Performance." *Journal of Applied Physiology* 100 (6): 2041–47.

Burgomaster, K. A., K. R. Howarth, S. M. Phillips, M. Rakobowchuk, M. J. Macdonald, S. L. McGee, and M. J. Gibala. 2008. "Similar Metabolic Adaptions During Exercise after Low Volume Sprint Interval and Traditional Endurance Training in Humans." *Journal of Applied Physiology* 586 (1): 151–60.

Burgomaster, K. A., S. C. Hughes, G. J. Heigenhauser, S. N. Bradwell, and M. J. Gibala. 2005. "Six Sessions of Sprint Interval Training Increases Muscle Oxidative Potential and Cycle Endurance Capacity in Humans." *Journal of Applied Physiology* 98 (6): 1985–90.

Campbell, B., R. B. Kreider, T. Ziegenfuss, P. La Bounty, M. Roberts, D. Burke, J. Landis, H. Lopez, and J. Antonio. 2007. "International Society of Sports Nutrition Position Stand: Protein and Exercise." *Journal of The International Society of Sports Nutrition* 4: 8.

Carpinelli, R. N., R. M. Otto. 1998. "Strength Training. Single versus multiple sets." *Sports Medicine* 26(2): 73-84.

CDC (Centers for Disease Control and Prevention). 2013. "Men and Heart Disease Fact Sheet." http://www.cdc.gov/dhdsp/data_statistics/fact_sheets/fs_men_heart.htm. Accessed 16 November 2017.

Chiang, Y., S. Lin, C. Cheng, and E. Liu. 2011. "Exploring Online Game Players' Flow Experiences and Positive Affect." *The Turkish Online Journal of Education Technology* 10 (1): 106–14.

Clark, N. 1997. *Nancy Clark's Sports Nutrition Guidebook*. Champaign, IL: Human Kinetics.

Cook, G. 2010. *Movement: Functional Movement Systems.*" Aptos, CA: On Target Publications.

Csikszentmihalyi, M. 1990. *Flow: The Psychology of Optimal Experience*. New York: Harper and Row.

Csikszentmihalyi, M. 2012. "Finding Flow [Review of the book Finding flow, by M. Csikszentmihalyi]." *Psychology Today*, Accessed 14 June 2016.

Csikszentmihalyi, M. 2013. *Creativity: Flow and the Psychology of Discover and Invention*. New York: Harper Collins Publishers.

Currell, K., and A. E. Jeukendrup. 2008. "Superior Endurance Performance with Ingestion of Multiple Transportable Carbohydrates." *Medicine & Science in Sports & Exercise* 40 (2): 275–81. https://doi.org/10.1249/mss.obo13e3181adf19. Accessed 14 June 2016.

Davis, J. M., N. L. Alderson, and R. S. Welsh. 2000. "Serotonin and Central Nervous System Fatigue: Nutritional Considerations." *American Journal of Clinical Nutrition* 72 (suppl): 573s–78s.

Davis, W. J., D. T. Wood, R. G. Andrews, L. M. Elkind, and W. B. Davis. 2008. "Concurrent Training Enhances Athlete's Strength, Muscle Endurance, and Other Measures." *Journal of Strength and Conditioning Research* 22(5): 1487-502.

De Villarreal, E. S., M. Izquierdo, and J. J. Gonzalez-Badillo. 2011. "Enhancing Jump Performance After Combined Vs. Maximal Power, Heavy-Resistance, and Plyometric Training Alone." *Journal of Strength and Conditioning Research* 25 (12): 3274–81. https://doi.org/10.1519/JSC.obo13e3182163085.

Donovan, C. M., and M. J. Pagliassotti. 2000. "Quantitative Assessment of Pathways for Lactate Disposal in Skeletal Muscle Fiber Types." *Medicine & Science in Sports & Exercise* 32 (4): 772–77.

Duncan, G. E., S. D. Anton, S. J. Sydeman, Newton, R. L Jr., J. A. Corsica, P. E. Durning, T. U. Ketterson, A. D. Martin, M. C. Limacher, and M. G. Perri. 2005. "Prescribing Exercise at Varied Levels of Intensity and Frequency; a Randomized Trial." *Achieves of Internal Medicine* 165 (20): 2362–69.

Farrell, S. W., G. M. Cortese, M. J. Lamonte, and S. N. Blair. 2007. "Cardiorespiratory Fitness, Different Measures of Adiposity, and Cancer Morality in Men." *Obesity* 15 (12): 3140–49.

Farrell, S. W., S. J. Fitzgerald, P. A. McAuley, and C. E. Barlow. 2010. "Cardiorespiratory Fitness, Adiposity, and All-Cause Mortality in Women." Medicine and Science in Sports and Exercise 42 (11): 2006–12. https://doi.org/10.1249/MSS.0b013e318df12bf.

Feinman, R. D., and E. J. Fine. 2004. "'A Calorie Is a Calorie' Violates the Second Law of Thermodynamics." *Nutrition Journal* 28 (3): 9. https://doi.org/10.1186/147s-2891-3-9.

Finke, P. and W. Finke. 2004. Marathoning, Start to Finish. Tualatin: wY'east Consulting.

Fontana, L., D. T. Villareal, E. P. Weiss, S. B. Racette, K. S. Steger-May, S. Klein, and J. O. Holloszy. 2007. "Calorie Restriction or Exercise: Effects on Coronary Heart Disease Risk Factors. A Randomized, Controlled Trial." *American Journal of Physiology-Endocrinology and Metabolism* 293 (1): E197–202.

Franklin, B. A. 2009. "Exercise Capacity: A Crystal Ball in Forecasting Future Health Outcomes?" *Physician and Sports medicine* 37 (4): 154–56. https://doi.org/10.3810/psm.2009.12.1754. Accessed 28 October 2017.

Friedlander, A. L., K. A. Jacobs, J. A. Fatter, M. A. Horning, T. A. Hagobian, T. A. Bauer, E. E. Wolfel, and G. A. Brooks. 2007. "Contributions of Working Muscle to Whole Body Lipid Metabolism are altered by Exercise Intensity and Training." *American Journal of Physiology-Endocrinology and Metabolism* 292 (1): E107-16. https://doi.org/10.1152/ajpondo.00148.

Gaesser, G. A., and G. A. Brooks. 1984. "Metabolic Bases of Excess Post-Exercise Oxygen Consumption: A Review." Medicine and Science in Sports and Exercise 16 (1): 29–43.

Giannoulis, M. G., P. H. Sonksen, M. Umpleby, L. Breen, C. Pentecost, M. Whyte, C. V. McMillan, C. Bradley, and F. C. Martin. 2006. "The Effects of Growth Hormone and/ or Testosterone in Healthy Elder Men: A Randomized Controlled Trial." *The Journal of Clinical Endocrinology and Metabolism* 91 (2): 477–84.

Gibala, M. 2009. "Molecular Responses to High-Intensity Interval Exercise." Applied Physiology, Nutrition, and Metabolism 34 (3): 428–32. https://doi.org/10.1139/H09-046.

Gibala, M. J., J. P. Little, M. Van Essen, G. P. Wilkin, K. A. Burgomaster, A. Safdar, S. Raha, and M. A. Tarnoolsky. 2006. "Short-term Sprint Interval Versus Traditional Endurance Training: Similar Initial Adaptions in Human Skeletal Muscle and Exercise Performance." *The Journal of Physiology* 575 (pt 3): 901–11.

Gibney, J., M. L. Healy, and P. H. Sönksen. 2007. "The Growth Hormone/Insulin-Like Growth Factor-I Axis in Exercise and Sport." *Endocrine Reviews* 28 (6): 603–24.

Gladden, L. B. 2000. "Muscle as a Consumer of Lactate." *Medicine & Science in Sports & Exercise* 32 (4): 764–71.

Goodpaster, B. H., S. W. Park, T. B. Harris, S. B. Kritchevsky, M. Nevitt, A. V. Schwartz, E. M. Simonsick, F. A. Tylavsky, M. Visser, and A. B. Newman. 2006. "The Loss of skeletal Muscle Strength, Mass, and Quality in Older Adults: The Health, Aging and Body Composition Study." *The Journals of Gerontology. Series A, Biological Sciences and Medical Sciences* 61 (10): 1059–64.

Google. 2014. "Define Lypolisis." Accessed 24 September 2017.

Goto, K., N. Ishii, S. Sugihara, T. Yoshioka, and K. Takamatsu. 2007. "Effects of Resistance Exercise on Lipolysis During Subsequent Sub Maximal Exercise." *Medicine and Science in Sports and Exercise* 39 (2): 308–15.

Gotshalk, L. A., C. C. Loebel, B. C. Nindl, M. Putukian, W. J. Sebastianelli, R. U. Newton, K.

Häkkinen, and W. J. Kraemer. 1997. "Hormonal Responses of Multiset Versus Single-Set Heavy-Resistance Exercise Protocols." *Canadian Journal of Applied Physiology* 22 (3): 244–55.

Guha, N., P. H. Sönksen, and R. I. Holt. 2009. "IGF-I Abuse in Sport: Current Knowledge and Future Prospects for Detection." *Growth Hormone and IGF Research* 19 (4): 408–11. https://doi.org/10.1016/j.ghir.2009.04.017.

Hargreaves, M. 2008. "Fatigue Mechanisms Determining Exercise Performance: Integrative Physiology Is Systems Biology." *Journal of Applied Physiology* 104 (5): 1541–42.

Hedley, G. 2012. "The Fuzz Speech by Dr. Gill Hedley." Retrieved from youtube.com, December 17, 2017.

Hoffman, J. R., N. A. Ratamess, J. Kang, M. J. Falve, and A. D. Faigenbaum. 2006. "Effect of Protein Intake on Strength, Body Composition and Endocrine Changes in Strength/Power Athletes." *Journal of The International Society of Sports Nutrition* 3 (2): 12–18. https://doi.org/10.1186/1550-2783-3-2-12.

Holm, I., M. A. Fosdahl, A. Friis, M. A. Risberg, G. Myklebust, and H. Steen. 2004. "Effect of Neuromuscular Training on Proprioception, Balance, Muscle Strength, and Lower Limb Function in Female Team Handball Players." *Clinical Journal of Sport Medicine* 14 (2): 88–94.

Hopkins, W. G. 2009. "The Improbable Central Governor of Maximal Endurance Performance." *Sports Science* 13:9–12.

Housch, D. J., T. J. Housh, and S. M. Rauge. 1990. "A Methodological Consideration for the Determination of a Critical Power and Anaerobic Work Capacity." *Research Quarterly for Exercise and Sport* 61 (4): 406–9.

Hsu, C., and H. Lu. 2003. "Why Do People Play On-Line Games? An Extended TAM with Social Influences and Flow Experiences." *Informational & Management* 41:853–68. https://doi.org/10.1016/jilm.2003.08.014.
    Ivy, J. L., P. T. Res, R. C. Sprague, and M. O. Widzer. 2003. "Effect of a Carbohydrate-protein Supplement on Endurance Performance During Exercise of Varying Intensity." International Journal of Sport Nutrition and Exercise Metabolism 13 (3): 382–95.

Jackson, S. A. 1992. "Athletes in Flow: A Qualitative Investigation of Flow States in Elite Figure Skaters." *Journal of Applied Psychology* 4 (2): 161–80. https://doi.org/10.1080/10413209208406459.

Jeukendrup, A. E. 1999. "Dietary Fat and Physical Performance." *Current Opinion in Clinical Nutrition and Metabolic Care* 2 (6): 521–26.

Jeukendrup, A. E. 2002. "Regulation of Fat Metabolism in Skeletal Muscle." *Annals of the New York Academy of Sciences* 967:217–35.

Jeukendrip, A. E., W. H. M. Saris, and A. J. M. Wagenmakers. 1998a. "Fat Metabolism during Exercise: A Review—Part I: Fatty Acid Mobilization and Muscle Metabolism. *International Journal of Sports Medicine* 19:231–44.

Jeukendrip, A. E. W. H. M. Saris, and A. J. M. Wagenmakers. 1998b. "Fat Metabolism during Exercise: A Review—Part II: Regulation of Metabolism and the Effects of Training. *International Journal of Sports Medicine* 19:293–302.

Jeukendrip, A. E., W. H. M. Saris, and A. J. M. Wagenmakers. 1998c. "Fat Metabolism during Exercise: A Review—Part III: Effects of Nutritional Interventions. *International Journal of Sports Medicine* 19:371–79.

Jeukendrup, A. E., J. J. Thielen, A. J. Wagenmakers, F. Brouns, and W. H. Saris. 1998d. "Effect of Medium-Chain Triacylglycerol and Carbohydrate Ingestion during Exercise on Substrate Utilization and Subsequent Cycling Performance." *American Journal of Clinical Nutrition* 67 (3): 379–404.

Johnson, C. 2013. *PR Pace: Strength & Performance Training for Distance Runners*. Boston: Lulu/Chris Johnson.

Kaleta, C., L. F. de Figueiredo, S. Werner, R. Guthke, M. Ristow, and S. Schuster. 2011. "In Silico Evidence for Gluconeogenesis from Fatty Acids in Humans." *PLoS Computational Biology* 7 (7): e1002116. https://doi.org/10.1371/journal.pcbi.1002116.

Kayser, B. 2003. "Exercise Starts and Ends in the Brain." *European Journal of Applied Physiology* 90:411–19.

Kemp, G. 2005. "Letters to the Editor." *Journal of Physiology-Regulatory, Integrative and Comparative Physiology* 289:895–901. https://doi.org/10.1152/ajpregu.00641.2004.

Kemp, G., D. Böning, R. Beneke, and N. Maassen. 2006. "Explaining pH Change in Exercising Muscle: Lactic Acid, Proton Consumption, and Buffering Vs. Strong Ion Difference." *Journal of Physiology-Regulatory, Integrative and Comparative Physiology* 291 (1): 235–37.

Kerksick, C., T. Harvey, J. Stout, B. Campbell, C. Wilborn, R. Kreider, D. Kalman, T. Ziegenfuss, H. Lopez, J. Landis, J. L. Ivy, and J. Antonio. 2008. "International Society of Sports Nutrition Stand: Nutrient Timing." *Journal of the International Society of Sports Nutrition* 5:17. https://doi.org/10.1186/1550-2783-5-17.

Knechtle, B., B. Baumann, A. Wirth, P. Knechtle, and T. Rosemann. 2010. "Male Ironman Triathletes Lose Skeletal Muscle Mass." *Asia Pacific Journal of Clinical Nutrition* 19 (1):91–97.

Koskek, M. A., L. S. Peseatello, R. L. Seip, T. J. Angelopoulos, P. M. Clarkson, P. M. Gordon, N. M. Moyna, P. S. Visich, R. F. Zoeller, P. D. Thompson, E. P. Hoffman, and T. B. Price. 2007. "Subcutaneous Fat Alterations Resulting from an Upper-body Resistance Training Progam." *Medicine and Science in Sports and Exercise* 39 (7): 1177–85.

Kotler, S. 2014. *The Rise of Superman: Decoding the Science of Ultimate Human Performance*. New York: Houghton Mifflin Harcourt Publishing Company.

Kowal, J., and M. S. Fortier. 2010. "Motivational Determinants of Flow: Contributions from Self- determination Theory." *The Journal of Social Psychology* 139 (3): 355–68. https://doi.org/10.1080/00224549909598391.

Kreider, R. B., M. Ferreira, M. Wilson, P. Grindstaff, S. Plisk, J. Reinardy, E. Cantler, and A. L. Almada. 1998. "Effects of Creatine Supplementation on Body Composition, Strength, and Sprint Performance." *Medicine & Science in Sports & Exercise* 30 (1): 73–82.

Kreider, R. B., C. D. Wilborn, L. Taylor, B. Campbell, A. L. Almada, R. Collins, M. Cooke, C. P. Earnest, M. Greenwood, D. S. Kalman, C. M. Kerksick, S. M. Kleiner, B. Leutholtz, H. Lopez, L. M. Lowery, R. Mendel, A. Smith, M. Spano, R. Wildman, D. S. Willoughby, T. N. Ziegenfuss, and J. Antonio. 2010. "ISSN Exercise & Sports Nutrition Review: Research & Recommendations." *Contemporary Issues in Health and Fitness* 7:7.https://doi.org/10.1186/1550-2783-7-7.

Krieger, J. W. 2009. "Single Versus Multiple Sets of Resistance Exercise: A meta-regression." *Journal of Strength and Conditioning Research* 23(6): 1890-901.

Kuipers, H., H. A. Keizer, F. Brouns, and W. H. M. Saris. 1987. "Carbohydrate Feeding and Glycogen Synthesis during Exercise in Man." *European Journal of Physiology* 410:652–56.

LaForgia, J., J. Dollman, M. J. Dale, R. T. Withers, and A. M. Hill. 2009. "Validation of DXA Body Composition Estimates in Obese Men and Women." *Obesity* (Silver Spring) 17 (4): 821–26. https://doi.org/10.1038/oby.2008.595.

Lambert, E. V., A. St. Clair Gibson, and T. D. Noakes. 2005. "Complex Systems Model of Fatigue: Integrative Homeostatic Control of Peripheral Physiological Systems during Exercise in Humans." *British Journal of Sports Medicine* 39:52–62.

Larson-Meyer, D. E., L. Redman, L. K. Heilbrenn, C. K. Martin, and E. Ravussin. 2010. "Caloric Restriction with or without Exercise: The Fitness Versus Fatness Debate." *Medicine and Science in Sports and Exercise* 42 (1): 152–59.

Lebrun, C. M. 1993. "Effect of the Different Phases of the Menstrual Cycle and Oral Contraceptives on Athletic Performance." *Sports Medicine* 16 (6): 400–30.

Lemon, P. W. 1991. "Protein and Amino Acid Needs of the Strength Athlete." *International Journal of Sport Nutrition and Exercise* 1 (2): 127–45.

Lindinger, M. I. 2008. "Rebuttal Letters." *Journal of Applied Physiology* 105:361–62. https://doi.org/10.1152/japplhysiol.00162.2008c.

Lindinger, M. I., J. M. Kowalchuk, and G. J. Heigenhauser. 2005. "Applying Physicochemical Principles to Skeletal Muscle Acid-Base Status." *Journal of Physiology-Regulatory, Integrative and Comparative Physiology* 289 (3): 891–94.

Little, J. P., A. Safdar, G. P. Wilkin, M. A. Tarnopolsky, and M. J. Gibala. 2010. "A Practical Model of Low-Volume High-Intensity Interval Training Induces Mitochondrial Biogenesis in Human Skeletal Muscle: Potential Mechanisms." *The Journal of Physiology* 588 (pt 6): 1011–22. https://doi.org/10.1113/jphysiol.2009.181743.

Lockwood, C. M., J. R. Moon, A. E. Smith, S. E. Tobkin, K. L. Kendall, J. L. Graef, J. T. Cramer, and J. R. Stout. 2010. "Low-calorie Energy Drink Improves Physiological Response to Exercise in Previously Sedentary Men: A Placebo-Controlled Efficacy and Safety Study." *Journal of Strength and Conditioning Research* 24 (8): 2227–38.

Lockwood, C. M., J. R. Moon, S. E. Tobkin, A. A. Walter, A. E. Smith, V. J. Dalbo, J. T. Cramer, and J. R. Stout. 2008. "Minimal Nutrition Intervention with High-protein/Low-carbohydrate and Low-fat, Nutrient-Dense Food Supplement Improves Body Composition and Exercise Benefits in Overweight Adults: A Randomized Controlled Trial." *Nutrition and Metabolism* (Lond) 21 (5): 11.

Loehr, L. R., W. D. Rosamond, C. Poole, A. M. McNeill, P. P. Chang, A. R. Folsom, L. E. Chambless, and G. Heiss. 2009. "Association of Multiple Anthropomtrics of Overweight and Obesity with Incident Heart Failure: The Atherosclerosis Risk in Communities Study." *Circa Heart Fail* 2 (1): 18–24. https://doi.org/10.1161/circheartfailure.108.813782.

Luscombe-Marsh, N. D., M. Noakes, G. A. Wittert, J. B. Keogh, P. Foster, and P. M. Clifton. 2005. "Carbohydrate-restricted Diets High in Either Monosaturated Fat or Protein Are Equally Effective at Promoting Fat Loss and Improving Blood Lipids." *The American Journal of Clinical Nutrition* 81 (4): 762–72.

Macedo, D. V., F. L. Lazarim, F. O. Catanho da Silva, L. S. Tessati, and R. Hohl. 2009. "Is Lactate Production Related to Muscular Fatigue? A Pedagogical Proposition using Empirical Facts." *Journal of Applied Physiology* 33 (4): 302–7.

Mäestu, J., A. Eliakim, J. Jürimäe, I. Valter, and T. Jürimäe. 2010. "Anabolic and Catabolic Hormones and Energy Balance of the Male Body Builders during the Preparation for the Competition." *Journal of Strength and Conditioning Research* 24 (4): 1074–81. https://doi.org/10.1519/JSC.obo13e3181cb6fd3.

Marcora, S. M. 2008. "Do We Really Need a Central Governor Model to Explain Brain Regulation of Exercise Performance?" *European Journal of Applied Physiology* 104 (5): 929–31.

Mårin, P., S. Holmång, L. Jönsson, L. Sjöstrom, H. Kvist, G. Holm, G. Lindstedt, and P. P. Björntorp. 1992. "The Effects of Testosterone Treatment on Body Composition and Metabolism in Middle-Age Obese Men." *International Journal of Obesity and Related Metabolic Disorders: Journal of the International Association for the Study of Obesity* 16 (12): 991–97.

Markovic, G. 2007. "Does Plyometric Training Improve Vertical Jump Height? A Meta-Analytical Review." *British Journal of Sports Medicine* 41 (6): 349–55. https://doi.org/10.1136/bjsm.2007.035133.

Markovic, G., I. Jukic, D. Milanovic, and D. Metidos. 2007. "Effects of Sprint and Plyometric Training on Muscle Function and Athletic Performance." *Journal of Strength and Conditioning Research* 21 (2): 543–49.

Martin, W. F., L. E. Armstrong, and N. R. Rodriguez. 2005. "Dietary Protein Intake and Renal Function." *Contemporary Issues in Health and Fitness* 2:25. https://doi.org/10.1186/1743- 7075-2-25.

Martinez-Lagunals, V., Z. Ding, J. R. Bernard, B. Wang, and J. L. Ivy. 2010. "Added Protein Maintains Efficacy of a Low-carbohydrate Sports Drink." *Journal of Strength and Conditioning Research* 24 (1): 48–59. https://doi.org/10.1519/JSC.0bo13e3181c32e2o.

McAuley, K. A., K. J. Smith, R. W. Taylor, R. T. McLay, S. M. Williams, and J. I. Mann. 2006. "Long-term Effects of Popular Dietary Approaches on Weight Loss and Features of Insulin Resistance." *International Journal of Obesity* 30 (2): 342–49.

McHugh, M. P., and C. H. Cosgrave. 2010. "To Stretch or Not To Stretch: The role of stretching in injury prevention and performance." *Scandinavian Journal of Medicine and Science in Sports* 20(2): 169-81.

McNamara, D. J. 2000. "The Impact of Egg Limitations on Coronary Heart Disease Risk: Do the Numbers Add Up?" *The Journal of the American College of Nutrition* 19 (5 suppl): 540s–48s.

Melanson, E. L., W. S. Gozansky, D. W. Barry, P. S. Maclean, G. K. Grunwald, J. O. Hill. 2009. "When Energy Balance Is Maintained, Exercise Does Not Induce Negative Fat Balance in Lean Sedentary, Obese Sedentary, or Lean Endurance-Trained Individuals." *Journal of Applied Physiology* 107 (6): 1847–56.

Meyertholen, E. 2014. The Krebs Cycle. Austin, TX: Austin Community College. http://www.austincc.edu/emeyerth/krebs.htm. Accessed 8 March 2016

Miller, M. G., J. J. Herniman, M. D. Ricard, C. C. Cheatham, and T. J. Michael. 2006. "The Effects of a 6-week Plyometric Training Program on Agility." *Journal of Sport Science and Medicine* 5 (3): 459–65.

Minderico, C. S., A. M. Silva, K. Keller, T. L. Branco, S. S. Martins, A. L. Palmeira, J. T. Barata, E. A. Carnero, P. M. Rocha, P. J. Teixeira, and L. B. Sardinha. 2008. "Usefulness of Different Techniques for Measuring Body Composition Changes during Weight Loss in Overweight and Obese Women." *British Journal of Nutrition* 99 (2): 432–41.

Moon, J. R., J. M. Eckerson, S. E. Tobkin, A. E. Smith, C. M. Lockwood, A. A. Waler, J. T. Cramer, T. W. Beck, and J. R. Stout. 2009a. "Estimating Body Fat in NCAA Division I Female Athletes: A Five-compartment Model Validation of Laboratory Methods." *European Journal of Applied Physiology* 105 (1): 119–30. https://doi.org/10.1007/500421-008-0881-9.

Moon, J. R., S. E. Tobkin, A. E. Smith, C. M. Lockwood, A. A. Walter, J. T. Cramer, T. W. Beck, and J. R. Stout. 2009b. "Anthropometric Estimations of Percent Body Fat in NCAA Division I Female Athletes: A 4-compartment Model Validation." *Journal of Strength and Conditioning Research* 23 (4): 1068–76. https://doi.org/10.1519/JSC.obo13e3181aa1cdo.

Myer, G. D., K. R. Ford, J. L. Brent, and T. E. Hewett. 2006a. "The Effects of Plyometric Vs. Dynamic Stabilization and Balance Training on Power, Balance, and Landing Force in Female Athletes." *Journal of Strength and Conditioning Research* 20 (2): 345–53.

Myer, G. D., K. R. Ford, S. G. McLean, and T. E. Hewett. 2006b. "The Effects of Plyometric Versus Dynamic Stabilization and Balance Training on Lower Extremity Biomechanics." *The American Journal of Sports Medicine* 34 (3): 445–55. The National Agricultural Library, The National Library of Medicine, The Library of Congress. February 27, 1998. "Joint Collection Development Policy: Human Nutrition and Food." http://www.nlm.nih.gov/pubs/cd_hum.nut.html#2. Accessed 7 June 2017.

Myers, T. W. 2011. *Anatomy Trains*. London: Urban & Fischer.

Nebelsick-Gullett, L. J., T. J. Housh, G. O. Johnson, and S. M. Bauge. 1988. "A Comparison between Methods of Measuring Anaerobic Work Capacity." *Ergonomics* 31 (10): 1413–19.

Nelson, R. J. 2005. *An Introduction to Behavioral Endocrinology*, Fourth Edition. Sunderland, MA: Sinauer Asssociates.

Neuromuscular Physiology Laboratory. n.d. "University of Florida Applied Physiology and Kinesiology College of Health and Human Performance." http://apk.hhp.ufl.edu/index.php/departments-centers/center-for-exercise-science-ces/neuromuscular-physiology-laboratory/. Accessed 3 September 2017.

Noakes, M., J. B. Keogh, P. R. Fosters, and P. M. Clifton. 2005. "Effect of an Energy-Restricted, High-Protein, Low-Fat Diet Relative to a Conventional High-Carbohydrate, Low-Fat Diet on Weight Loss, Body Composition, Nutritional Status, and Markers of Cardiovascular Health in Obese Women." *The American Journal of Clinical Nutrition* 81 (6): 1298–306.

Noakes, T. D. 2007. "The Central Governor Model of Exercise Regulation Applied to the Marathon." *Sports Medicine* 37 (4–5): 374–77.

Noakes, T. D., and F. E. Marino. 2009. "Point: Counterpoint: Maximal Oxygen Uptake Is/is Not Limited by a Central Nervous System Governor." *Journal of Applied Physiology* 106 (1): 338–39. https://doi.org/10.1152/japplphysiol.90844.2008.

Noakes, T. D., and A. St. Clair Gibson. 2004. "Logical Limitations to the "Catastrophe" Models of Fatigue during Exercise in Humans." *British Journal of Sports Medicine* 33 (4): 302–7.

Noakes, T. D., A. St. Clair Gibson, and E. V. Lambert. 2004. "From Catastrophe to Complexity: A Model Novel of Integrative Central Neural Regulation of Effort and Fatigue during Exercise in Humans." *British Journal of Sports Medicine* 38 (5): 648–49.

Nordmann, A. J., A. Nordmann, M. Briel, U. Keller, Yancy, W. S Jr., B. J. Brehm, and H. C. Bucher. 2006. *Archives of Internal Medicine* 166 (3): 285–93.

Norton, L. E., and D. K. Layman. 2006. "Leucine Regulates Translation Initiation of Protein Synthesis in Skeletal Muscle after Exercise." *Journal of Nutrition* 136 (2): 533s–37s.

Nybo, L., E. Sundstrup, M. D. Jakobsen, M. Mohr, T. Hornstrup, L. Simonsen, J. Bülow, Randers, M. B., J. J. Nielsen, P. Aagaard, and P. Krustrup. 2010. "High-intensity Training Versus Traditional Exercise Interventions for Promoting Health." *Medicine and Science in Sports and Exercise* 42 (10): 1951–58. https://doi.org/10.1249/MSS.obo13e3181d.

Ojeda, S. R. and J. B. Griffin. 2000. *Textbook of Endocrine Physiology*. 4th ed. Oxford [Oxfordshire]: Oxford University Press.

Oosthuyse, T., and A. N. Bosch. 2010. "The Effect of the Menstrual Cycle on Exercise Metabolism: Implications for Exercise Performance in Eumenorrhoeic Women." *Sports Medicine* 40 (3): 207–27. https://doi.org/10.2165/112170 90-000000000-00000.

Orpana, H. M., J. M. Berthelot, M. S. Kaplan, D. H. Feeny, B. McFarland, and N. A. Ross. 2010. "BMI and Mortality: Results from a national longitudinal study of Canadian adults." *Obesity* 18(11): 214-8.

Ostoji´c, S. M., M. Stojanovi´c, and Z. Ahmetovi´c. 2010. "Vertical Jump as a Tool in Assessment of Muscular Power and Anaerobic Performance." *Medicinski Pregled* 63 (5–6): 371–75.

Pánics, G., A. Tállay, A. Pavlik, and I. Berkes. 2008. "Effect of Proprioception Training on Knee Joint Position Sense in Female Team Handball Players." *British Journal of Sports Medicine* 42 (6): 472–76. https://doi.org/10.1136/bjsm.2008.046516.

Poole, D. C. 1986. "Letter to the Editor-in-Chief." *Medicine and Science in Sports and Exercise* 18:703–4.

Poortmans, J. R., and O. Dellalieux. 2000. "Do Regular High Protein Diets Have Potential Health Risks on Kidney Function in Athletes?" *International Journal of Sport Nutrition and Exercise Metabolism* 10 (1): 28–38. https://doi.org/10.1249/mss.obo13e31815adf19.

Potteiger, J. A., R. H. Lockwood, M. D. Haub, B. A. Dolezal, K. S. Almuzaini, J. M. Schroeder, C. J. Zebas. 1999. "Muscle power and fiber characteristics following 8 weeks of plyometric training." *Journal of Strength and Conditioning Research* 13 (3): 275–79.

Redman, L. M., L. K. Heilbronn, C. K. Martin, A. Alfonso, S. R. Smith, E. Ravussin, and Pennington Calerie Team. 2007. "Effect of Calorie Restriction with or without Exercise on Body Composition and Fat Distribution." *The Journal of Clinical Endocrinology and Metabolism* 92 (3): 865–72.

Robergs, R. A., F. Ghiasvand, and D. Parker. 2004. "Biochemistry of Exercise-induced Metabolic Acidosis." *Journal of Applied Physiology* 287 (3): 502–16.

Robergs, R. A., F. Ghiasvand, and D. Parker. 2005. "Lingering Construct of Lactic Acidosis." *Journal of Physiology-Regulatory, Integrative and Comparative Physiology* 289:904–10. https://doi.org/10.1152/ajpregu.00117.2005.

Roberts, C. K., M. Katiraie, D. M. Croymans, O. O. Yang, and T. Kelesidis. 2013. "Untrained Young Men Have Dysfunctional HDL Compared with Strength-Trained Men Irrespective of Body Weight Status." *Journal of Applied Physiology* 115 (7): 1043–49.

Roberts, F. 2000. "Respiratory Physiology." Physiology 12 (11): 1–3.

Roberts, M. D., V. J. Dalbo, S. E. Hassel, and C. M. Kerksick. 2009. "The Expression of Androgen- regulated Genes before and after a Resistance Exercise bout in Younger and Older Men." *Journal of Strength and Conditioning Research* 23 (4): 1060–67. https://doi.org/10.1519/JSC.obo13e3181a59bdd.

Romero-Corral, A., V. M. Montori, V. K. Somers, J. Korinek, R. J. Thomas, T. G. Allison, F. Mookadam, and F. Lopez-Jimenez. 2006. "Association of Bodyweight with Total Mortality and with Cardiovascular Events in Coronary Artery Disease: A Systematic Review of Cohort Studies." *Lancet* 368 (9536): 666–78.

Ross, A., and M. Leveritt. 2001. "Long-term Metabolic and Skeletal Muscle Adaptions to Short-Sprint Training: Implications for Sprint Training and Tapering." *Sports Medicine* 31 (15): 1063–82.

Rowland, T. W. 2011. *Athlete's Clock: How Biology and Time Affect Sport Performance.* Champaign, IL: Human Kinetics.

Roy, B. D. 2008. "Milk: The New Sports Drink? A Review." *Journal of the International Society of Sports Nutrition* 5:15. https://doi.org/10.1186/1550-2783-5-15.

Salekzamani, Y., A. Shirmohammadi, M. Rahbar, K. Shakouri, and F. Nayebi. 2011. "Association between Human Body Composition and Periodontal Disease." *ISRN Dentistry* 2011:863847. https://doi.org/10.5402/2011/863847.

Santos, D. A., A. M. Silva, C. N. Matias, D. A. Fields, S. B. Heymsfield, L. B. Sardinha. 2010. "Accuracy of DXA in Estimating Body Composition Changes in elite Athletes using a Four-component Model as the Reference Method." *Nutrition and Metabolism* (Lond) 22 (7): 22. https://doi.org/10.1186/1743-7075-7-22.

Sattler, F. R., C. Castaneda-Sceppa, E. F. Binder, E. T. Schroeder, Y. Wang, S. Bhasin, M. Kawakubo, Y. Stewart, K. E. Yarasheski, J. Ulloor, P. Colletti, R. Roubenoff, and S. P. Azen. 2009. "Testosterone and Growth Hormone Improve Body Composition and Muscle Performance in Older Men." *The Journal of Clinical Endocrinology and Metabolism* 94 (6): 1991–2001. https://doi.org/10.1210/jc.2008-2338.

Sawyer, B. J., J. R. Blessinger, B. A. Irving, A. Weltman, J. T. Patrie, and G. A. Gaesser. 2010. "Walking and Running Economy: Inverse Association with Peak Oxygen Uptake." *Medicine and Science in Sports and Exercise* 42 (11): 2122–27. https://doi.org/10.1249/MMS.obo13e3181de2da7.

Sedliak, M., T. Finni, S. Cheng, W. J. Kraemer, and K. Häkkinen. 2007. "Effect of Time-of-Day-Specific Strength Training on Serum Hormone Concentrations and Isometric Strength in Men." *Chronobiology International* retrieved from tandfonline.com, November 9, 2017.

Sedliak, M., T. Finni, S. Cheng, M. Lind, and K. Häkkinek. 2009. "Effect of Time-of-Day-Specific Strength Training on Muscular Hypertrophy in Men." *Journal of Strength and Conditioning Research* 23(9): 2451-7.

Sedliak, M., T. Finni, J. Peltonen, and K. Häkkinen. 2008. "Effect of Time-of-Day-Specific Strength Training on Maximum Strength and EMG Activity of The Leg Extensors in Men." *Journal of Sports Sciences* 26(10): 1005-14.

Shaw, B. S., I. Shaw, and G. A. Brown. 2009. "Comparison of Resistance and Concurrent Resistance and Endurance Training Regimes in The Development of Strength." *Journal of Strength and Conditioning Research* 23(9): 2507-14.

Shepard, R. 2009. "Is It Time to Retire the Central Governor?" *Sports Medicine* 39:709–21.

Shernoff, D. J., M. Csikszentmihalyi, B. Shneider, E. S. Shernoff. 2003. Student engagement in high school classrooms from the perspective of flow theory. School Psychology Quarterly, 18(2), 158–76.

Silva, A. M., D. A. Fields, A. L. Quitério, and L. B. Sardinha. 2009. "Are Skinfold-based Models Accurate and Suitable for Assessing Changes in Body Composition in Highly Trained Athletes?" *Journal of Strength and Conditioning Research* 23 (6): 1688–96. https://doi.org/10.1519/JSC.obo13e3181b3foe4.

Sonntag, W. E., L. J. Forman, N. Miki, and J. Meiters. 1982. "Growth Hormone Secretion and Neuroendocrine Regulation." In *Handbook of Endocrinology*, edited by G. H. Gass and H. M. Kaplan, 35–39. Boca Raton, FL: CRC Press.

Spriet, L. L, R. A. Howlett, and G. J. Heigenhauser. 2000. "An Enzymatic Approach to Lactate Production in Human Skeletal Muscle during Exercise." *Medicine & Science in Sports & Exercise* 32 (4): 756–63.

Stallnect, B., F. Dela, and J. W. Helge. 2007. "Are Blood Flow and Lipolysis in Subcutaneous Adipose Tissue Influenced by Contractions in Adjacent Muscles in Humans?" American Journal of Physiology. *Endocrinology and Metabolism* 292 (2): 394–99.

Stein, G. L., J. C. Kimiecik, J. Daniels, and S. A. Jackson. 1995. "Psychological Antecedents of Flow in Recreational Sport." *Personality & Social Psychology Bulletin* 21 (2): 125–35. https://doi.org/10.11771014616729521003.

Støren, O., J. Helgerud, E. M. Støa, and J. Hoff. 2008. "Maximal Strength Training Improves Running Economy in Distance Runners." *Medicine and Science in Sports and Exercise* 40(6): 1087-92.

Sui, x., M. J. LaMonte, J. N. Laditka, J. W. Hardin, N. Chase, S. P. Hooker, and S. N. Blair. 2007. "Cardiorespiratory Fitness and Adiposity as Morality Predictors in Older Adults." *JAMA* 298 (21): 2507–16. https://doi.org/10.1001/jama.298.21.2507.

Swart, J., R. P. Lamberts, M. I. Lambert, A. St. Clair Gibson, E. V. Lambert, J. Skowno, and T. D. Noakes. 2009. "Exercising with Reserve: Evidence that the Central Nervous System Regulates Prolonged Exercise Performance." *British Journal of Sports Medicine* 43 (10): 782–88.

Symons, T. B., S. E. Schutzler, T. L. Cocke, D. L. Chinkes, R. R. Wolfe, and D. Paddon-Jones. 2007. "Aging Does Not Impair the Anabolic Response to a Protein-Rich Meal." *The American Journal of Clinical Nutrition* 86 (2): 451–56.

Szulc, P., F. Munoz, F. Marchand, R. Chapurlat, and P. D. Delmas. 2010. "Rapid Loss of Appendicular Skeletal Muscle Mass Is Associated with Higher All-Case Mortality in Older Men: The Prospective MINOS Study." *The American Journal of Clinical Nutrition* 91 (5): 1227–36. https://doi.org/10.3945/ajcn. 2009.28256.

Taylor, K., J. M. Sheppard, H. Lee, and N. Plummer. 2009. "Negative Effects of Static Stretching Restored When Combined with A Sport Specific Warm-up Component." *Journal of Science and Medicine in Sport* 12(6): 657-661.

Tricoli, V., L. Lamas, R. Carnevale, and C. Ugrinowitsch. 2005. "Short-term Effects on Lower-body Functional Power Development: Weightlifting Vs. Vertical Jump Training Programs." *Journal of Strength and Conditioning Research* 19 (2): 433–37.

Tucker, R. and J. Dugas. 2009. The Runner's Body. New York, NY: Rodale Inc.

Uchida, M. C., B. T. Crewther, C. Ugrinowitsch, R. F. Bacurau, A. S. Moriscot, and M. S. Aoki. 2009. "Hormonal Responses to Different Resistance Exercise Schemes of Similar Total Volume." *Journal of Strength and Conditioning Research* 23 (7): 2003–8. https://doi.org/10.1519/JSC.obo13e3181b73bf7.

Van Vonderen, K. E., and W. Kinnally. 2012. "Media Effects on Body Image: Examining Media Exposure in the Broader Context of Internal and Other Social Factors." *American Communication Journal* 14 (2): 41–57.

Walts, C. T., E. D. Hanson, M. J. Delmonico, L. Yao, M. Q. Wang, and B. F. Hurley. 2008. "Do Sex or Race Differences Influence Strength Training Effects on Muscle or Fat?" *Medicine & Science in Sports & Exercise* 40 (4): 669–76.

Wang, Z. M., P. Deurenberg, S. S. Guo, A. Pietrobelli, J. Wang, R. N Pierson Jr., and S. B. Hymsfield. 1998. "Six-compartment Body Composition Model: Inter-method Comparisons of Total Body Fat Measurement." *International Journal of Obesity and Related Metabolic Disorders* 22 (4): 329–37.

Weir, J. P., T. W. Beck, J. T. Cramer, and T. J. Housh. 2006. "Is Fatigue All in Your Head? A Critical Review of the Central Governor Model." *British Journal of Sports Medicine* 40 (7): 573–86.

Weir, J. P., D. A. Keefe, J. F. Eaton, R. T. Augustine, and D. M. Tobin. 1998. "Effect of Fatigue on Hamstring Coactivation during Isokinetic Knee Extensions." *European Journal of Applied Physiology* 78 (6): 555–59.

Weir, J. P., A. L. McDonough, and V. J. Hill. 1996. "The Effects of Joint Angle on Electromyographic Indices of Fatigue." *European Journal of Applied and Occupational Physiology* 73 (3–4): 387–92.

Weltman, A., J. Y. Weltman, R. Schurrer, W. S. Evans, J. D. Veldhuis, and A. D. Rogol. 1985. "Endurance Training Amplifies the Pulsatile Release of Growth Hormone: Effects of Training Intensity." *Journal of Applied Physiology* 72 (6): 2188–96.

Westerblad, H., D. G. Allen, and J. Lannergren. 2002. "Muscle Fatigue: Lactic Acid or Inorganic Phosphate the Major Cause?" *News in Physiological Sciences* 17:17–21.

Weyand, P. G., D. B. Sternlight, M. J. Bellizzi, and S. Wright. 2000. "Faster Top Running Speeds are Achieved with Greater Ground Forces Not More Rapid Leg Movement." *Journal of Applied Physiology* 89(5): 1991-9.

Widdowson, W. M., M. L. Healy, P. H. Sönksen, and J. Gibney. 2009. "The Physiology of Growth Hormone and Sport." *Growth Hormone & IGF Research* 19 (4): 308–19. https://doi.org/10.1016/j.ghir.2009.04.023.

Wilkinson, D. J., N. J. Smeeton, and P. W. Watt. 2010. "Ammonia Metabolism, the Brain and Fatigue, Revisiting the Link." *Progress in Neurobiology* 91 (3): 200–19. https://doi.org/10.1016/j.pneurobio.2010.01.012.

Williams, P. T., and P. D. Thompson. 2013. "Walking Versus Running for Hypertension, Cholesterol, and Diabetes Mellitus Risk Reduction." *Arteriosclerosis, Thrombosis, and Vascular Biology* 33 (5): 1085–91. https://doi.org/10.1161/ATVBAHA.112.300878.

Willoughby, D. S., and L. Taylor. 2004. "Effects of Sequential Bouts of Resistance Exercise on Androgen Receptor Expression." *Medicine and Science in Sports & Exercise* 36 (9): 1499–509.

Wilson, G. J., A. J. Murphy, and A. Giorgi. 1996. "Weight and Plyometric Training: Effects on Eccentric and Concentric Force Production." Canadian Journal of Applied Physiology 21 (4): 301–15.

Wilson, G. J., R. U. Newton, A. J. Murphy, and B. J. Humphries. 1993. "The Optimal Training Load for the Development of Dynamic Athletic Performance." *Medicine and Science in Sports & Exercise* 25 (11): 1279–86.

Wisløff, U., C. Castagna, J. Helgerud, R. Jones, and J. Hoff. 2004. "Strong Correlation of Maximal Squat Strength with Sprint Performance and Vertical Jump Eight in Elite Soccer Players." *British Journal of Sports Medicine* 38:285–88. https://doi.org/10.1136/bjsm.2002.002071.

Withers, R. T., J. LaForgia, R. K. Pillans, N. J. Shipp, B. E. Chatterton, L. G. Schultz, and F. Leaney. 1998. "Comparisons of Two-, Three-, and Four-compartment Models of Body Composition Analysis in Men and Women." *Journal of Applied Physiology* 85 (1): 238–45.

Wolf, C. n.d. "Assessment and Corrective Exercise Strategies for Improved Shoulder Function." *Ideafit.* retrieved from ideafit.com, December 26, 2017.

Zebis, M. K., J. Bencle, L. L. Andersen, S. Døssing, T. Alkjar, S. P. Magnusson, M. Kjaer, and P. Aagaard. 2008. "The Effects of Neuromuscular Training on Knee Joint Motor Control during Side Cutting in Female Elite Soccer and Handball Players." *Clinical Journal of Sport Medicine* 18 (4): 329–37. https://doi.org/10.1097/JSM.obo13e31817f3e35.

Zehnder, M., E. R. Crist, M. Ith, K. J. Acheson, E. Pouteau, R. Kreise, R. Trepp, P. Diem, C. Boesch, and J. Decombaz. 2006. "Intramyocellular Lipid Stores Increased Markedly in Athletes after 1.5 Days Lipid Supplementation and Are Utilized during Exercise in Proportion to Their Content." *European Journal of Applied Physiology* 98 (4): 341–54.

Zehnder, M., M. Ith, R. Kreis, W. Saris, U. Boutellier, and C. Boesch. 2005. "Gender-specific Usage of Intramyocellular Lipids and Glycogen during Exercise." *Medicine & Science in Sports & Exercise* 37 (9): 1517–24.

Zierath, J. 2011. "A Workout Can Change Your DNA." *Cell Metabolism.*

Index

W

Walking · 17, 175, 177
warm up · 15
water · 14, 18, 24, 38, 45, 94, 96, 139

weight · 12, 13, 20, 30, 31, 37, 42, 43, 47, 49, 50, 51, 61, 66, 68, 70, 73, 79, 84, 85, 86, 101, 102, 112, 135, 136, 140
weight machines · 13
weightlifting · 49, 61
work capacity · 50, 89
Workout · 177

About the Author

Christopher P. Johnson is a human performance expert combing sport and exercise science with personal and team leadership. Coach Johnson is an officer in the Army National Guard, doctoral student (ABD), Boston Marathon qualifier, former sponsored athlete, college lecturer, and co-founder of Boston Strength & Conditioning. When he is not helping others improve to reach their goals, he is hiking in the mountains or snorkeling in the ocean. Chris resides in Newton, Ma with his wife Stephanie.

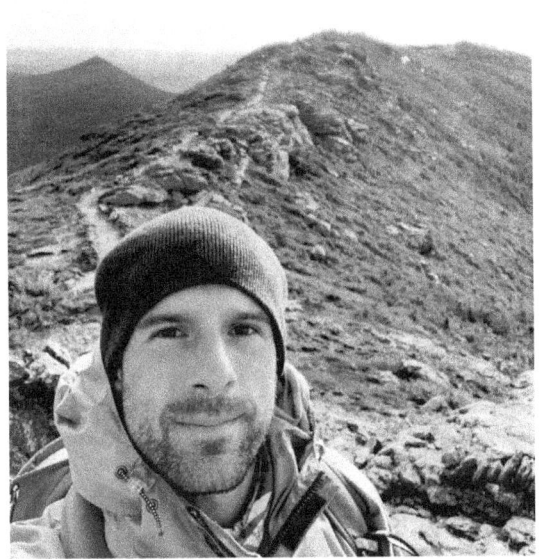

To learn more about Chris visit www.improvewithchris.com

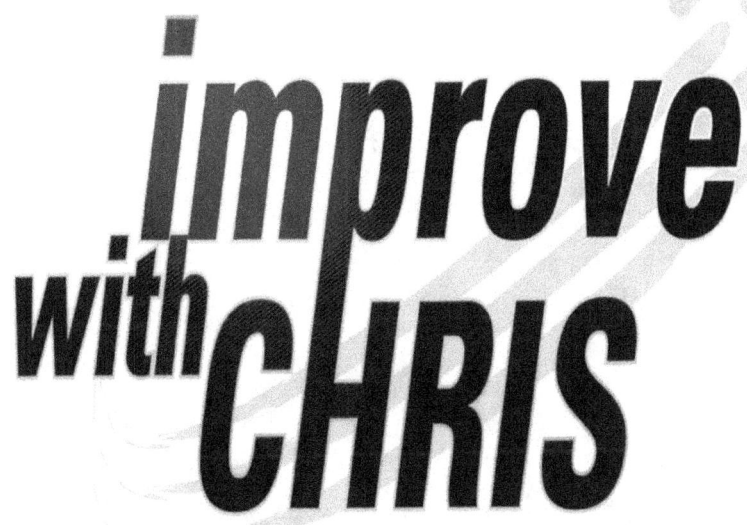